A STUDY COURSE
IN
HOMOEOPATHY

A STUDY COURSE IN HOMOEOPATHY

by
PHYLLIS SPEIGHT

The C.W. Daniel Company Ltd.
1 Church Path, Saffron Walden, Essex, England

3rd IMPRESSION 1986
New Edition 1991

ISBN 0 85207 250 3

Printed in Great Britain by
Hillman Printers
(Frome) Ltd
Frome, Somerset

CONTENTS

INTRODUCTION

In presenting this course of instruction on Homoeopathy, I am attempting the very difficult task of condensing a philosophy and art of medicine into a comparatively simple form whereby those who are truly interested in the Art of Healing may be encouraged to study man and the ills that afflict him.

To do this I have tried to give the basic points necessary for an understanding of this vast subject but I emphasize that text books must be obtained for study and reference. These will be recommended as we go along.

Hahnemann the founder of Homoeopathy said: 'There are no diseases but only sick persons' and when this is considered it will be realised that every experience and every bit of knowledge that can be garnered will be of essential value to those who would treat Homoeopathically.

The unqualified practitioner can and does do very useful work especially in these days when qualified Homoeopathic Physicians are few, but it must be remembered that the layman is always limited by the absence of a hospital training and the experience that can be gained thereby; and the fact that his physical examination of the patient can only be on the surface of the body. At no time should the layman make an internal examination of a patient but be prepared to call in the advice of a qualified physician if a particular case appears to warrant it.

The course of 12 lessons leads the student from a knowledge of the basic principles of Homoeopathy to an understanding of their application to sick people in relation to acute and chronic affections. Some of the most important Homoeopathic remedies are outlined. The method of case-taking and suggestions for questioning the patient are detailed in the effort to help the beginner to collate his facts accurately.

Only by such care and precise work can the real value of Homoeopathic treatment become an established fact. I would ask every student to remember that in undertaking to treat any

1

sick person, however simple the affection or injury may be, he is taking on a real responsibility. Homoeopathy is a great study and not to be undertaken lightly, but it well repays the efforts and sacrifices it entails.

Restoration to health and happiness becomes apparent when the correct remedy is administered according to the laws laid down by Hahnemann.

Each lesson is accompanied by a short question paper, which the student should answer when he feels he has mastered the particular lesson. Specimen answers are given at the end of the book.

Lesson 1

PRINCIPLES OF HOMOEOPATHY

'Truth for which all the eager world is fain,
which makes us happy, lies for evermore
Not buried deep but lightly covered o'er,
By the wise Hand that destined it for men'

What is Homoeopathy

The followers of the Law of Similars believe that disease is intimately associated with the life of the individual and is a result of internal concealed causes; that pathological tissue changes are the *end*-results of the disease, and if cure is to be effected the *whole individual man* must be treated.

No two persons are exactly alike, each individual being made up of particular characteristics by which he is distinguished from his neighbour — the form of the body, colour of the hair and eyes, height, gait, abilities and so on. Similarly no two persons react in the same way to a particular medical treatment. Those who believe in the Law of Similars, therefore, use a system of medicine by which their remedies are prescribed strictly according to the individual requirements of each sick person.

Homoeopathy is based on the Law of Similars. Indeed, the word itself is from the Greek-Homoion meaning 'Similar', and Pathos meaning 'Disease'. The Law of Similars means that a remedy which creates symptoms and conditions in a *healthy* person will cure a *sick* person manifesting similar symptoms. This can be summed up in the dictum Similia Similibus Curentur.

The Founding of Homoeopathy

'An illness is caused by similar means and similar means can cure men of illness, e.g. the same agent brings about strangury when it is not present, and does away with it, when it is. Coughing, like strangury, is caused and is made to disappear by

3

the same means. Vomiting is stopped by being made to vomit.'
Hippocrates 460-377 B.C.

Homoeopathy was founded by Dr Samuel Hahnemann (1755-1843). Receiving his degree of M.D. in 1779, he soon earned the reputation of being a brilliant chemist and one of the most distinguished physicians in Germany at that time. Yet as his experience grew, he became more and more dissatisfied with the current medical practice which consisted largely of bleeding and purging the patient, or forcing him to swallow large draughts of drug mixtures supposedly good for the particular complaint suffered.

After a few years experience of these methods Hahnemann felt that the cure of disease, or even the restoration of health, was so problematical that he was compelled to give up his practice, and earned his living subsequently by making translations of works on chemistry and medicine. In 1790 he was translating an English Materia Medica into German and found that he could not agree with the explanation of the action of Cinchona Bark (Quinine) in the cure of ague.

During his medical training Hahnemann spent two years in the marshy lands of Hungary where he came into contact with malaria (ague fever) which was rife in the district. When he left he had a thorough knowledge of this disease and the treatment to cure it. Now he decided to test Cinchona on himself. Let us take up the story in his own words:

'For the sake of experiment, I took for several days four quentschen (drachms) of good Cinchona twice a day. My feet, the tips of my fingers, etc., first became cold, and I felt tired and sleepy; then my heart began to beat, my pulse became hard and quick, I got an insufferable feeling of uneasiness, a trembling (but without rigor), a weariness in all my limbs, then a beating in my head, redness of the cheeks, thirst; in short, all the old symptoms with which I was familiar in Ague appeared one after the other. Also, those particularly characteristic symptoms which I was wont to observe in Agues-obtuseness of the senses, a kind of stiffness in all the limbs, but especially that dull disagreeable feeling which seems to have its seat in the periosteum of all the bones of the body, — these all put in an appearance. This paroxysm lasted each time for two or three hours, and came again afresh whenever I repeated the dose, not otherwise. I left off, and became well.'

Note that when Hahnemann ceased taking the drug the symptoms disappeared, yet when he repeated his experiment identical symptoms returned. It was a genuine drug effect. *That which could cure ague could also produce symptoms similar to those of ague.*

Opponents of Homoeopathy have sought to discredit this initial experiment of Hahnemann's, stating that Cinchona has no real power of causing in the healthy such a fever as that 'imagined' by him, and that its action in the cure of ague is not on the body but on the minute organisms of which Malaria consists. Yet over the years, abundant proof of the true action of Cinchona has been found, agreeing in all details with Hahnemann's experiment. Later you will read how all drugs have an individual and characteristic effect on the body, and it is sufficient here to state that the experiment which Hahnemann undertook to find the true action of Cinchona gave him his initial insight into the Law of Similars.

Continuing his story: 'I now commenced to make a collection of the morbid phenomena which different observers had from time to time noticed as produced by medicines introduced into the stomachs of healthy individuals, and which they had casually recorded in their works. But as the number of these was not so great, I set myself diligently to work to test several medicinal substances on the healthy body and see the carefully observed symptoms they produced corresponded wonderfully with symptoms of the morbid states they would easily and permanently cure.'

For six years Hahnemann continued his experiments and studies before tentatively making his findings known. He then wrote an essay in a current medical journal in which he stated: 'Every powerful medicinal substance produces in the human body a peculiar kind of disease — the more powerful the medicine, the more peculiar, marked and violent the disease. We should imitate nature, which sometimes cures a chronic disease by superadding another, and employ in the disease we wish to cure that medicine which is able to produce another very similar artificial disease, and the former will be cured, similia similibus.'

In 1810 Hahnemann produced 'The Organon of Rational Medicine' in which he gives a full dissertation on the theory of his method, together with detailed instructions for the examination of patients, proving of drugs, and for the selection of remedies according to the Homoeopathic principle.

In the introduction he set out his newly discovered rules of healing as follows: 'Hitherto, Diseases of man were *not* healed *in a rational way* or according to fixed principles, but rather according to very varied curative purposes, amongst others, according to the palliative rule: contraria contrariis curentur. In contrast to this is the truth, the real way of healing, which I am pointing out in this volume: In order to cure gently, quickly and lastingly, choose in every case of illness a remedy which can itself arouse a similar malady to that which it is to cure (similia similibus curentur)!

'Hitherto nobody has taught this Homoeopathic method of healing. But if it is truth who is prescribing this method, then even if She has been disregarded for thousands of years, it is to be expected that traces of Her Immortal influence can be discovered in all epochs. And so it is.'

He then traces various glimmerings throughout history of the action of Homoeopathic Law. He did not pretend to be the first and only discoverer of this method of healing, but stressed the fact that 'Till now nobody has *taught* this Homoeopathic way of healing, nobody has *carried it out*.'

It should be noted that, in all, six editions of The Organon were completed by Hahnemann. Progressively over the years, as his knowledge of pure drug actions in the treatment of disease grew, so additions and amendments were made to the original treatise. But the basic, fundamental structure of *The Organon* remained, and remains today, for anyone to follow.

Throughout this course we shall be making constant references to *The Organon* and to Hahnemann's subsequent writings in order that you may obtain an insight into the Master's philosophy. He makes clear at the outset what is required to practice the healing art and it is fitting that we should, in this first lesson, thoroughly understand Hahnemann's injunctions: 'The doctor's highest and *only* calling is to make sick men well, to cure, as it is called.'

If the physician clearly perceives what is to be cured in diseases, that is to say, in every individual case of disease (knowledge of disease, indication); if he clearly perceives what is curative in medicines, that is to say, in each individual medicine (knowledge of medicinal powers); and if he knows how to adapt, according to clearly-defined principles, what is curative in medicines to what he has discovered to be un-doubtedly morbid in the patient, so that recovery must ensue — to adapt it, as well in respect to the suitableness of the medicine most appropriate according to its mode of action to the case before him (choice of the remedy, the medicine indicated), as also in respect to the exact and proper period for repeating the dose; if, finally, he knows the obstacles to recovery and is aware how to remove them, so that the restoration may be permanent; then he understands how to treat judiciously and rationally, and he is a true practitioner of the healing art.'

The Four Fundamental Laws
1. The Law of Similars
2. The single remedy.
3. The minimum dose.
4. The direction of cure. (This will be dealt with later)

On these laws the whole application of Homoeopathy as an art of medicine rests, but added to this is the necessity for an accurate knowledge of each patient and the true observation of him and the manifestations of his sickness.

We have already explained the Law of Similars and we must now consider the second and third laws, the single remedy and the minimum dose.

While the first law (The Law of Similars) must always apply, Hahnemann stated: 'The day of true knowledge of medicines and of the true healing art will dawn when physicians shall trust the cure of complete cases of disease to a *single* medicinal substance, and when . . . they will employ for the extinction and cure of a case of disease, whose symptoms they have investi-gated, *one single* medicinal substance, whose positive effects they have ascertained, which can show among these effects a group of symptoms very similar to those presented by the case of disease. . .'

And again: 'In no case of healing is it necessary (and for that reason alone it is unpermissible) to use more than one simple medicinal substance on the patient at a time. It is difficult to understand why there should be the slightest doubt about whether it is more natural and more rational in a case of illness to use only one simple medicinal substance of known qualities

at a time or a mixture of several different ones. In Homoeopathy, the only true, simple and rational science of healing, it is
absolutely unpermissible to give the patient two different medicinal substances at the same time.'

The necessity for the third law of Homoeopathic medicine
was brought about by Hahnemann's observations that when
prescribing the similar remedy in the then recognised dosage,
the disease was initially aggravated. From this he deduced that
the dose prescribed was too large and proceeded, therefore, to
dilute the remedy on strictly mathematical lines. He found that
by this method he not only avoided the aggravations of the
disease, but the efficiency of the medicine was increased.

'The spiritual power of medicine achieves its object not by
quantity but by quality.'

'The suitability of a medicine for any given case of disease
does not depend on its accurate homoeopathic selection alone,
but likewise on the proper size, or rather smallness of the dose.'

'A medicine which when given by itself in a sufficiently large
dose to a healthy individual produces a definite effect, that is, a
number of its own peculiar symptoms, preserving its own
tendencies, will be able to produce them even in the smallest
dose . . . for curative purposes incredibly small doses are sufficient . . . if instead of smaller and smaller doses, increasingly
large ones were given, then (after the original disease has disappeared) there arise merely medicinal symptoms, a kind of
artificial and unnecessary disease. . . How much the sensitiveness of the body towards medicinal stimuli increases the illness
can only be appreciated by the accurate observer. Especially
when the disease has become very serious, this surpasses all
belief. . . On the other hand, it is just as true as it is remarkable that even the most robust people, who are suffering from a
chronic disease, notwithstanding their abundant physical
strength, as soon as they are given the medicine positively
helpful in their chronic disease, experience just as great an impression from the smallest possible dose, as if they were suckling
babes.'

From these quotations you will realise that the mathematical
reduction of the amount of medicine introduces an entirely new
approach in dealing with sickness and disease.

The reduction of the dose (potentization or dynamisation)
will be dealt with in greater detail later. It should be noted that

Hahnemann applied his rules in the treatment of all sick persons and invariably found that he could cure when other methods failed.

Summary
1. Homoeopathy is the art of medicine based on the Law of Similars.
2. Homoeopathy was founded and developed by Samuel Hahnemann, a German physician and chemist, who collated his theories in a book called 'The Organon'.
3. The four Laws of Homoeopathy:
    1. The Law of Similars; 2. The single remedy;
    3. The minimum dose; 4. The direction of cure.

The keen student must obtain a copy of *The Principles and Art of Cure by Homoeopathy* by Dr Herbert A. Roberts and Chapters I and II should be studied carefully.

TEST PAPER No. 1

These questions should be answered only when the student feels confident that the lesson has been mastered. There should be no reference to books as this would defeat the object.

1. What is the basic fundamental Law of Homoeopathy?
2. It is maintained that Homoeopathy treats the individual patient. State briefly why this is so.
3. Why is it advisable to use single remedies only?

Lesson 2

WHAT IS DISEASE?

The two dominant schools of medicine look upon disease, its nature, cause and cure, from totally different standpoints.

The allopathic or orthodox school regards disease as a positive material entity, caused by the invasion of the organism from the outside, by some obnoxious foreign element or elements, which are to be antidoted, destroyed or expelled in the most direct manner possible. This purely material view of disease finds its culmination in the so-called 'germ-theory'.

In contrast, the homoeopath looks upon disease as a dynamic disturbance of that harmonious relation, which in health exists between the material body and the *vital force* which animates that body.

Paragraph 16 of the 'Organon' teaches us the very important lesson that our sickness comes from dynamic disturbances and that, therefore, our curative agents must have a similar dynamic quality.

The material evidence of chronic disease manifesting in the physical body is but the result of long continued derangement of the vital force, perhaps perverted during the lifetime of an individual, and incited by an inherited tendency which again may have been in many generations of his ancestors.

This is one of the greatest stumbling blocks to students of Homoeopathy. It is so difficult to grasp that it is the *man* himself who is sick, as well as a part, or an organ. Serious consequences are often the result when the importance of this law is not fully appreciated, and attempts are made to cure disease by removing an affected organ, part or tumour, without first attacking it through its symptomatology. The vital force that has been brought to work in an orderly manner by the use of the indicated remedies, will often remove all kinds of symptoms in a way that is surprising.

No organ functions completely independently of any other

organ, nor does it become diseased independently of itself, for the reason that it depends on other organs for some part of its life, and in turn the functions performed by it are necessary for the well being of other organs in the human economy.

One organ cannot become diseased without its functions becoming first impaired and thereby disturbing the normal functions of other organs, to a greater or less extent, through improper stimulation. It is therefore plain that the whole man is sick also, and that the totality of symptoms is an index of the diseased condition and a guide for treatment.

Organic diseases are changes in the structure of the organs themselves. This condition must have had a beginning which was of a functional nature. This state is not completely revealed by examination but through the sensations and functions of those parts of the organism felt by the patient and observed by the physician. These are *morbid symptoms*. 'In no other way can it make itself known.'

Therefore, disease is first a 'change of state' ultimating in disfunction of vital processes, to be soon followed by morbid cell growth or tissue change.

This is probably the most difficult point in Homoeopathic philosophy to accept. Unless the student has a clear understanding that the vital processes of the patient must be taken into consideration as well as the part or organ that is sick, then cure cannot be achieved.

The Cause of Disease

Disease does not 'just happen'. Its origin may be from an event or series of events, extending over many years. Sometimes the cause is an inherited constitutional fault, or it may be a progressive accumulation of toxic material in the organisms created by defective elimination. Other causative factors are bad hygiene, over-indulgence in bad habits, over-eating or malnutrition.

Ailments often appear as a result of a severe mental or physical shock such as grief, prolonged anxiety, or great disappointment.

It will be seen, therefore, that the fundamental causes of disease spring from two main sources:

1. Inherited — the type of constitution.

2. Acquired — direct contamination, physical or emotional shocks, hygiene and dietetic lapses.

Inherited Causes. These are being dealt with at length later as they are most important in our treatment of chronic ailments.

Acquired Causes. Direct contamination covers the endemic and epidemic diseases. Endemic is the term applied to disease which exists in particular localities or amongst certain races. For example cholera is an endemic disease of certain parts of Asia. Epidemic is the term applied to a disease which affects a large number of people in a particular locality at one time. This type of disease is, therefore, infectious from person to person.

Many epidemic diseases occur at certain regular seasons. For example, typhoid fever begins to show itself in August, increases during the autumn months and gradually decreases during the winter. Scarlatina and diphtheria are autumnal complaints. Whooping cough usually occurs during the spring. Measles produces two epidemics, one in mid-summer and one in December.

Physical and emotional shocks which may be the root cause of a patient's disorder will be revealed when the patient is questioned by the practitioner; from this questioning any hygienic or dietetic lapses should also become evident.

It should be noted that all curable diseases created by these causes can be removed, or greatly modified, by correct Homoeopathic treatment. In simple or acute cases, the correct remedy produces an almost instantaneous effect. A demonstration of this rapid action will be seen when Arnica is given for shock and bruising from an accident.

In chronic cases one may have to wait weeks, or even months, but improvement will follow providing the disease has not ultimated itself in gross pathological changes.

The Proving of Remedies

Hahnemann spent a great deal of his life, aided by some fifty keen fellow workers (mostly doctors) in testing, or 'proving' remedies as to their subversive possibilities in regard to human sensations and health, and he most carefully recorded his findings in the simple language of the provers, and according to a definite schema which renders them readily accessible. These drug provings formed the nucleus of the Homoeopathic

Materia Medica.

Hahnemann himself says 'After a considerable number of simple drugs have been tested in this manner on healthy persons and after every element or symptom of disease which these drugs are capable of producing has been carefully noted and faithfully recorded, we shall then possess a true Materia Medica.'

He goes on 'It will consist of a collection of genuine, pure and undeceptive effects of simple drugs; it will be a code of nature. . . These records will contain and represent in similitude the homoeopathic elements of natural diseases hereafter to be cured by these means. In other words, these records will contain lists of symptoms of *artificial diseases;* and these afford the only true specific means for a certain and permanent cure of *similar natural diseases.*'

'There is therefore no other possible way in which the peculiar effects of medicines on the health of individuals can be accurately determined: there is no sure, and no more natural way of accomplishing this, than to administer the different medicines experimentally, in moderate doses, to healthy persons, in order to ascertain what changes, symptoms and signs each produces on the healthy body and mind; that is to say, what disease-elements they can, or tend to produce. For as has been shown, all the curative power of medicines lies in their power to alter the health of man; and is revealed by observations on the latter.'

And so we come back once more to The Law of similars — when again in Hahnemann's own words we read:

'The day of true knowledge of medicines and of the true healing art will dawn when physicians shall trust the cure of complete cases of disease to a single medicinal substance and when they will employ for the extinction and cure of a case of disease, whose symptoms they have investigated, one single medicinal substance whose positive effects they have ascertained, which can show among these effects a group of symptoms very similar to those presented by the case of disease.'

(A point that needs clarification is that only one remedy may be given as a prescription but as symptoms change it will be necessary to follow the first remedy with another, and so on).

The mere investigation of drugs, without any law for their subsequent application in disease, is of poor and limited usefulness. It is Hahnemann alone, who in his Law of Similars, established for all time the relationship between drug and disease, i.e. between drug-disease and natural disease; proving that the one can neutralise and extinguish the other; and so made medicine not only scientific but practical.

In Hahnemann's words 'A fundamental principle of the Homoeopathic physician (which distinguishes him from every physician of all the older schools) is this, that he never employs for any patient a medicine, whose effects on the healthy human has not been previously and carefully proved and thus made known to him. To prescribe for the sick on mere conjecture of some possible usefulness for some similar disease, or from hear-say, "that a remedy has helped in such and such a disease"—such conscienceless venture the philanthropic homoeopathist will leave the Allopath.'

'These morbid disturbances called forth by drugs in the healthy body, must be accepted as the only possible revelation of their inherent curative power. Through them only we are able to discover what capacity of producing disease — and hence what capacity of curing disease — is possessed by each individual drug.'

Every medicine has its own peculiar action on the human body, unlike that of any other and therefore medicines must be tested on healthy individuals in order to obtain an accurate knowledge of their powers; the provers must be very trust-worthy and they must be able to describe their sensations accurately. Medicines must be tested on males and females in order that any alterations in the health of the sexual sphere may be revealed. All the symptoms of a medicine will not appear in one person, or all at once.

All the various symptoms from the drug proving are subse-quently collected and collated and written down in the form of the schema and this constitutes the record in the Materia Medica.

Chapter XV of Roberts' *Principles and Art of Cure by Homoeo-pathy* on Drug Proving should be studied.

The Study of Remedies

The student must become familiar with as many remedies as possible and there is no substitute for hard work to achieve this end.

Knowledge of the mental symptoms is essential as the inner-most part of man is the most important (his loves, desires etc.).

The characteristics of each remedy must be mastered, for instance, you would not give Sulphur as a chronic remedy to a patient who is fastidious to a degree about his home and his person; neither would you give Arsenicum Alb., to a patient with slovenly habits.

Modalities must be memorised; in other words, aggravations or ameliorations from weather conditions, motion, heat, touch, position, certain foods etc.

The marked desires and aversions, aggravations and ameliorations should be etched on the mind of the student; those which affect the patient as a whole and those which modify the affected part. These are sometimes contradictory as in Arsenicum Alb., where the patient himself is worse cold but his head is better for cold air.

The student should note the locality of the body to which the remedy especially applies — not only the organ influenced by the remedy should be learned but also the tissues — e.g. Bryonia is suitable for inflammation of serous membranes, where Belladonna is rarely so.

Throughout this course we give details of a number of remedies and these should be studied in several Materia Medicas and the student should equip himself from the following:

Clarke's *Dictionary of Practical Materia Medica* which is the fullest as regards the number of remedies. This is a large work in 3 volumes with a section at the beginning giving the characteristic symptoms. It is a very important addition to the library.

Kent's *Lectures on Homoeopathic Materia Medica* should be obtained by every student as, although informal in style, this author gives wonderful mental pictures of approximately 300 remedies.

Tyler's *Homoeopathic Drug Pictures* also, should be on the bookshelf of the keen student. One hundred and twenty five remedies are covered and in addition to the basic information Dr. Tyler quotes from several sources and illustrates the points she is making by short case histories from her records.

There is, of course, nothing like going to the fountain head for information and Hahnemann's *Materia Medica Pura,* the prime source of the subject is packed with a mass of symptoms.

There are many more which, no doubt, will be collected as time goes on but too long a list may confuse the student, however, one more is worthy of note here and that is Hering's *Condensed Materia Medica* which covers over 400 remedies.

In each case *do read the Preface* before proceeding. Each author writes to explain his method of presentation.

ACONITUM NAPELLUS

Characteristics
Anxiety; Unreasonable Fears; Terror; Restlessness. Pains, which are to the patient intolerable. Suddenness of ailments; worse cold dry winds.

Mind:	Tension, emotional and mental as shown in fright or fear and its consequences. Unreasonable fears of something that will happen. Restlessness, tossing about in agony — (the fear helping to make him restless).
Head:	Vertigo worse exposure to sun. Headaches through exposure to sun generally, better in open air; worse in warm room. Headache worse drinking.
Eyes:	Affections worse dry cold winds. Inflammations from cold, injury, dust and surgical operations.
Nose:	Fluent coryza, frequent sneezing, dripping of clear hot water; worse cold dry winds.
Face:	Red and flushed but turns pale on rising up from bed. Dry burning heat without sweat (fever).
Mouth:	Dryness; unquenchable thirst. Everything tastes bitter except water. Tongue white or yellow-white; prickling or burning sensation.
Throat:	Pain and deep redness of affected part; scraping, tingling sensation with burning and prickling, chiefly on swallowing. Acute inflammation of throat.
Respiratory:	Continual tickling of larynx with constant desire to cough. Cough worse eating and drinking; short and dry; particularly at night..
Chest:	Oppression of chest worse ascending. Cough

	worse every inspiration. After cough, tingling in chest. Cough worse cold dry winds.
Limbs:	Pains tearing and cutting accompanied with tingling and numbness; patient very restless. Motion aggravates pains in muscles, joints and stiffness. All these pains are worse cold dry winds.
Modalities:	Worse cold dry winds; worse in evening; worse lying on left side; worse in warm room or for warm covering. Better uncovering — kicks off the clothes.

NUX VOMICA

Characteristics

Over sensitive; every harmless word offends. Sensitive to every little noise. Great heat, whole body burning hot, especially face red and hot, yet patient cannot move or uncover in the least without feeling chilly. Frequent and ineffectual desire to defaecate or passing but small quantities of faeces at each attempt. Awakens tired and weak and generally worse (many complaints).

Mind:	Angry and very irritable and peevish. Excitable, fiery temper. Breaks out in acts of violence.
Head:	Burning pain in forehead after eating and on waking; pressing pain in forehead worse cold air. Headaches from mental exertion, chagrin or anger. Headaches worse in open air; on waking; after eating; from abuse of coffee, spirits, on stooping, from light, noise, moving eyes, high living etc.
Nose:	Coryza a.m. better open air. Coryza from sitting on cold stones or steps. Stopped up nose.
Stomach:	After eating, sour taste. Pressure in stomach an hour or so after eating with tightness about waist, must loosen clothing. Confused in mind 2—3 hours after eating, epigastrium bloated with pressure as from stone in stomach. Patient says 'If I could only vomit I would feel better'. The patient is worse for coffee, alcoholic drinks,

	debauchery, abuse of drugs, business anxiety, sedentary habits, too high living etc.
Rectum:	Constipation but constant desire for stool, passing but small quantities of faeces at each attempt. The harder one strains the harder it is to pass stools.
Back:	Sore bruised beaten feeling in lumbar region. Lumbago worse lying in bed. Must sit up to turn over in bed. Backache worse 3—4 a.m.
Chill:	Chilly — cannot get warm however many extra clothes or bedcovers he has — worse uncovering.
Modalities:	Better heat (except head); unbroken sleep. (very chilly patient). Worse around 4 a.m. and worse from losing sleep. Worse mental effort and dry cold and windy weather.

Nux Vomica acts best when given at night.

Nash says 'More stress may be placed upon the cause of the stomach, liver and abdominal complaints for which Nux Vom., is the remedy. For instance, coffee, alcoholic drinks, debauchery, abuse of drugs, business anxiety, sedentary habits, broken rest from long night-watching, too high living etc.'

TEST PAPER No. 2

These questions should be answered only when the student feels confident that the lesson has been mastered. There should be no reference to books as this would defeat the object.

1. What are the causes of disease?

2. Why are provings made only on healthy persons?

3. Give five characteristic indications of Aconitum.

Lesson 3

THE LAW OF DIRECTION OF CURE

Bodily reactions to the similar remedy occur in a definite direction, viz:

Cure takes place from above downward; from within outward; from an important organ to a less important organ; symptoms disappear in the reverse order of their appearance, the first to appear being the last to disappear.

Let us consider these axioms.

1. *From above downward.* When the correct remedy has been administered it is seen that the pain in the shoulder will travel down the arm to the hand, or from the hip to the foot.

2. *From within outward.* Crises of elimination often occur, e.g. an eruption breaks out on the skin, there is an increased flow of urine, or the symptoms of a severe cold become apparent. These manifestations should never be interferred with. Nature is attempting to rid the system of disease attacking the deeper organs by bringing the bye-products to the surface — the cure taking place from the important organ such as the heart, the kidneys, etc., to the less important, the bladder, the skin, etc.

3. *Symptoms disappear in the reverse order of their appearance.* Measles can be taken as an example, the cough coming first and departing last, the rash coming last and departing first. In cases of chronic disease it is found that the patient will retrace the road along which his disease has travelled and he will experience again the various ailments from which he has suffered until he gets back to the conditions from which his disease started.

We observe from this law that following the administration of the remedy, if some unexpected crisis occurs, such as is mentioned above, or the patient suddenly finds that he has produced symptoms of a complaint he had long ago, this is excellent and we must allow the curative process to continue undisturbed. *On no account should further medicine be given at this point.* Read Chapter 10 of Roberts' *The Principles & Art of Cure by Homoeopathy.*

The Preparation of Homoeopathic Remedies

'To serve the purposes of Homoeopathy, the spirit-like medicinal powers of crude substances are developed to an unparalleled degree by means of a process which was never attempted before, and which causes medicines to penetrate the organism, and thus to become more efficacious and remedial. It is applicable even to those substances which, in their crude state, do not evince the least medicinal effect upon the human body.' — The Organon.

Homoeopathic dosage is in conformity with the law of physics that Action and Reaction are equal and opposite. All remedies have this dual action in the body — a primary physiologic, or toxic (harmful) action, and a secondary therapeutic or curative action. The possible good effect of any remedy is directly proportional to its power to derange the healthy human organism. Hence those remedies which are the greatest poisons when administered in a large dose become the greatest medicines when administered in a minute dose.

When Hahnemann realised that the aggravation of disease was due to the strength of a remedy he systematically reduced it by a method which has continued to the present day. This method is known as potentisation and may be described as follows:

In a phial containing 99 drops of alcohol 1 drop of the strong tincture of a remedy is added and the whole *vigorously shaken.* This proportion of 1 in 100 is called the first centesimal dilution or 1c. Of this solution 1 drop is added to another phial containing 99 drops of alcohol — this is again *shaken,* thus giving the second centesimal dilution (2c) and this procedure is repeated until the required potency is achieved.

Insoluble substances are ground up with sugar of milk in the same proportions as above, in a porcelain mortar, and again the 1 in 100 potency is obtained. One grain of this with 99 grains of sugar of milk ground up gives the 2c potency. When the third centesimal or one in a million has been reached, then the substance becomes soluble in alcohol or water and potencies may be followed along the lines for liquid medicines.

Since Hahnemann's time another scale has also been used, whereby the proportion of remedy to alcohol is 1 in 10 only. This is the decimal scale and remedies made up in this scale have X after the number of the potency — e.g. 3x, 6x.

The following extract from Hahnemann's *Chronic Diseases* will be of interest:

'The alteration which is effected in the properties of natural substances, especially medicinal substances, either by triturating or shaking them in conjunction with a non-medicinal powder or liquid, is almost marvellous. This discovery is due to Homoeopathy. Besides this alteration of their medicinal properties, the homoeopathic mode of preparing medicines produces an alteration in their chemical properties. Whereas, in their crude form, they are insoluble either in water or alcohol, they become entirely soluble, both in water and alcohol, by mean of this homoeopathic transformation. This discovery is invaluable to the healing art.'

'The brown-black juice of a sea-insect, Sepia, which was formerly used only for painting and drawing, is soluble in water only, while in its unprepared form. When homoeopathically prepared by trituration, it becomes soluble in alcohol. . .'

'Lycopodi pollen floats in alcohol and on the surface of water, without either of these substances having the least effect upon the drug; Lycopodium in its crude state, on being introduced into the stomach, is both tasteless and inactive. Trituration makes it soluble in both alcohol and water, and develops such a powerful medicinal action in the drug that its use requires great care.'

'Who ever found marble, or the shell of an oyster soluble in water or alcohol? This mild calcarea, as well as baryta carbonica and magnesia, becomes perfectly soluble by means of the homoeopathic trituration, which, moreover develops their medicinal powers to an astonishing degree.'

The Potency to Use

Hahnemann made this observation on potencies: 'Experience proves that the dose of a homoeopathically selected remedy cannot be reduced so far as to be inferior in strength to the natural disease, and to lose its power of extinguishing and curing at least a proportion of the same, provided that this dose, immediately after having been taken, is capable of causing a slight intensification of symptoms of the similar natural disease.'

The 'slight intensification of symptoms' refers to the aggravation of symptoms which follows administration of the similar remedy, and should be noted as being a direct effect caused by the similarity of the remedy symptoms to the disease symptoms, and to the potency used.

Following are the rules which will guide you in deciding the potency to use:

1. Be sure that the remedy selected is a near similar (or similimum).

2. When the remedy has been selected it should be given in the appropriate potency until no appreciable improvement in the patients condition is observable. If the patients condition is not completely cured and the symptoms remain the same, the potency may then be advanced, i.e. if the first prescription was given in the 6th the second can be advanced to the 30th — but under no circumstances should remedies be changed unless the symptoms warrant it.

3. Low potencies only should be used when the disease has caused a great amount of organic change. For example, in an advanced case of arthritis a high potency would probably cause a severe and most painful aggravation. Similarly a sharp reaction is usually observed in chronic skin complaints when a high potency is given.

4. The higher potencies should only be prescribed where there is little or no organic change, and the indication for the remedy very definite. These are not generally for the beginner or layman to use as the reactions resulting can present grave complications and even endanger life.

5. In general, use the lower potencies in acute conditions (6th—12th) and the higher potencies (30th—200th) in chronic conditions. It will be found that one dose alone is often sufficient to bring about a marked improvement in a chronic case which will continue for some considerable

time. The dose should, therefore, *not* be repeated until there is an indication of definite relapse.

Note most carefully any warning given in the Materia Medicas about certain remedies and their effects in particular complaints. For example, Drosera and Silica in respiratory affections and Sulphur in its relation to incipient T.B.

Read Chapters 12 and 13 of Roberts' *The Principles & Art of Cure by Homoeopathy*

In this, and following lessons, some general information is given regarding the skin, bowels, vomiting, urine, appetite, thirst, tongue, expectoration, pain, the pulse, temperature and respiration.

These general hints help to determine, in some cases, the cause of sickness.

The Skin and Perspiration

In health the skin is soft and slightly moist. There should be no roughness, tension, or cracking of the surface.

Normal perspiration is a means of excreting waste products from the body and amounts to considerably over one pint in twenty four hours. It is a slightly acid fluid containing a very small percentage of solids made up chiefly of salts, a little fatty material and a small amount of urea, the substance which the kidneys secrete in large amounts. When the action of the kidneys is defective the skin tends to compensate by excreting urea and other waste products in increased quantities. This will be recognised by offensive odour, or by the staining of linen.

Excessive perspiration, unless produced by healthy exercise, will be observed in:

1. A critical phase in an acute condition. This is an evidence of bodily reaction to the disease and will be observed by an improvement in the condition which will follow.

2. An early phase of disease when it is actually a symptom of the disease, e.g. in various stages of fevers. There is no relief following a sweat of this nature.

Localised sweating, e.g. on the head, is found in certain conditions. In children a profuse perspiration around the head and neck when asleep indicates a tendency to rickets.

Severe night-sweats are a strong indication of the tubercular constitution, and where a history of such sweats is elicited it is always advisable to call in a qualified Homoeopathic Physician.

In an acute condition, however, the critical sweat mentioned in (1) above is evidenced by the whole body surface perspiring at the same time, with a relaxation of tension, return to normal pulse-rate, and immediate relief of other symptoms — (see notes on temperatures).

Vomiting

This is brought about by the concerted action of abdominal and stomach muscles controlled by nervous centres in the brain, or solar plexus. It may be caused by irritation of the nerves of the stomach or other related organs, or by strong impressions of an unpleasant nature such as an ugly sight or smell. Interference with the sense of balance also has the same effect, such as travelling in a moving vehicle, or in sea sickness.

Vomiting of watery fluid usually indicates disturbances to the brain, i.e. brain tumours, but is also found in other conditions such as vomiting in the early months of pregnancy.

Mucus, when vomited in considerable amount in strings, and especially when sour in taste and brought up in the morning, is a sign of catarrh of the stomach.

Bile may be brought up by any long-continued attack of vomiting, after the contents of the stomach has been expelled and retching still continues. Usually the bile is golden-yellow.

Vomiting of blood usually indicates some ulceration in the oesophagus or stomach, and may be red in colour but usually resembles coffee grounds.

In all cases of vomiting the concomitant symptoms must be taken into consideration in order to determine the possible cause.

BELLADONNA

Characteristics

Belladonna stands for REDNESS — HEAT — INTENSE BURNING. Great general sensitiveness (to light, motion, noise or jar). Pains come and go suddenly. Worse lying down.

Mind: Rage: Delusions of imaginary animals etc., worse 3 p.m. until midnight.

Head: Confusion. Pains throbbing, pulsating, darting, pressive, boring, burning. Worse movement, worse jar of bed, worse weight of hair and worse wetting hair.

Eyes: Heat and burning; heaviness of eye-lids; dilated pupils, bloodshot; staring; red.

Nose: Fluent coryza of one nostril alternating with stoppage. Pain as if bruised, sometimes with burning.

Face: Burning heat, glowing redness and bloated appearance. Purple, red, hot.

Mouth: Great dryness without thirst. Accumulation of saliva, thick viscid.

Throat: Very red and dry. Scraping and shooting pain principally on swallowing, sometimes extending to ears. Great dryness and burning. Inflammation and swelling and sensation of a lump; constant inclination to swallow.

Abdomen: Tenderness aggravated by the least jar in walking or stepping, or even a jar against the bed or chair upon which the patient sits or lies; pressure downwards as if the contents of the abdomen would issue through the vulva — worse mornings. With this pressure there is often associated a pain in the back 'as if it would 'break'.

Respiratory: Tenacious mucus in chest; catarrh with cough, coryza, hoarseness. Loss of voice. Great soreness in larynx. Dry spasmodic cough.

Skin: Very red and hot; burns the hand that touches it; sweats on covered parts.

Modalities: Symptoms worse afternoon; 3 p.m., 11 p.m. and after midnight. Worse touch, motion, noise, draughts, cold applications, lying down, uncovering the head.

Kent says 'The Belladonna throat burns like coals of fire; the inflamed tonsils burn like fire. The skin burns like fire to the patient and is intensely hot to the Doctor... Put your hand on a

Belladonna patient and you want to suddenly withdraw it; the heat is so intense.'

Remember Belladonna then, in inflammatory or congestive conditions — whatever disease name they may have, such as appendicitis or pneumonia — if the characteristic symptoms of Belladonna are present this remedy will cure.

Violence is another characteristic. Dr. Tyler says 'Violence runs through Belladonna, violence and suddenness. We associate Belladonna in our minds with sudden violence — violent pain, violent headache, violent throbbing, violent delirium, violent mania, violent starts and twitchings, violent convulsions.' She goes on 'The typical Belladonna picture is unmistakable when you meet it; the bright red face, the dilated pupils, the burning skin, the throbbing pains, the intolerance of pressure and jar. These call for Belladonna whatever the disease.'

Belladonna is one of our best remedies in the diseases of children — the child is often well one minute and sick the next.

Dr. Nash said that he considered Belladonna one of the trio of delirium remedies with Hyocyamus and Stramonium, and Belladonna may also be called pre-eminently a head remedy. He says 'In most cases when this remedy is indicated, head symptoms predominate.'

'The blood seems to be rushing to the head. The head is hot while the extremities are cool. The eyes are red and blood-shot. The face is also red, almost purple red.'

ARNICA

Characteristics
Sore, bruised feeling all over. REMEMBER SORENESS AND BRUISING — ARNICA. Head and face hot; body and extremities cold. Recent and remote affections from injuries.

Removes physical soreness and bruising from soft parts but it also removes shock caused by accidents and injuries.

This remedy is suited to persons who are extremely sensitive to mechanical injuries and who feel the effects of them long afterwards, and where SORENESS is attached to any symptom.

Mind: Patient says he is not ill and demands that the doctor be sent away.

Head: Pressing pain especially in forehead. Pain as if nail were driven into brain. Sore bruised feeling. Pains worse midnight.

Limbs: Sore and bruised feeling worse movement. Body sore as if pounded, extremely sore to touch the bed, chair or couch on which the patient sits or lies feels hard as a rock, causing him to seem very restless and change position often to get off the sore parts on which he lies. Backache worse breathing deeply.

Skin: Black and blue — bruising. Crops of small boils.

Sleep: Sleepless and restless when physically overtired.

Modalities: Worse cold, damp weather; motion and exertion aggravates. Better lying down.

HYPERICUM

The characteristic of the Hypericum wounds is that they are very sensitive to touch.

Injuries to parts rich in sentient nerves; especially fingers, toes, matrices of nails.

Lacerations when the intolerable pain shows nerves are severely involved.

Always modifies and sometimes arrests ulceration and sloughing.

Puncture wounds feel very sore (from treading on nails; rat-bites etc.). Prevents lockjaw.

Wounds from crushing, as mashed fingers, especially tips. Great nervous depression following wounds, and effects of shock or fright.

Neck and back. After a fall slightest motion of arms or neck cries; cervical vertebrae very sensitive to touch. Entire spine tender. Violent pain and inability to walk or stoop after a fall on coccyx.

Nerves. Prevents lockjaw from wounds in soles of feet, fingers or palms of hands. Lacerated pains excruciating.

Pains. Lightning pains and electric shocks — if this is allowed to go on there is every likelihood of the patient ending up with tetanus.

TEST PAPER No. 3

These questions should be answered only when the student feels confident that the lesson has been mastered. There should be no reference to books as this would defeat the object.

1. Describe briefly the law of Direction of Cure.

2. In general when should the higher potencies be used.

3. Name the characteristics of Belladonna.

4. Give two examples when Arnica should be given.

5. Give one example when Hypericum should be given.

Lesson 4

CHRONIC DISEASES

We have dealt with the basic principles of Homoeopathy as laid down by Hahnemann. With a knowledge of these principles much good work can be done. Yet Hahnemann went a great deal further in the latter part of his life, supplementing his earlier work by making a deep study of Chronic Diseases.

First let us understand the difference between an acute and a chronic disease.

Acute:

Those diseases originating from dietary indiscretions, deficient hygiene, physical agents, or bacterial infections. There is a period of progress and a period of decline, and there is always a tendency towards recovery. An example of this can be seen in typhoid, which is due to an acute poison having an evolution ending in recovery or death. Acute diseases, then, run a definite course and are of limited duration.

Chronic:

Those diseases caused by infection from various sources having a period of progress but NO period of decline. The vital force alone is unable to extinguish these diseases — hence they cease only with the death of the patient, there being no tendency whatever to recovery unless cured by proper treatment. Syphilis is an example, its manifestations changing over the years of the patient's life, but ever striking deeper towards the vital organs.

Hahnemann, in his practice, observed that the homoeopathic remedies he was then using were successful in curing the ailments of many patients, yet after a period of time some returned with similar symptoms stronger than before. The disease was in fact progressing.

He states 'It was a continually repeated fact that the non-

29

venereal chronic diseases, after being time and again removed
homoeopathically by the remedies fully proved up to the
present time, always returned in a more or less varied form and
with new symptoms, or reappeared annually with an increase of
complaints. This fact gave me the first clue that the homoeopathic physician . . . has not only to combat the disease presented before his eyes . . . but that he has always to encounter only
some separate fragment of a more deep-seated *original* disease.'

'He, therefore, must first find out as far as possible the *whole
extent* of all the accidents and symptoms belonging to the
unknown primitive malady before he can hope to discover one
or more medicines which may homoeopathically cover the
whole of the original disease by means of its peculiar symptoms. . .'

'But that the original malady sought for must be also of a
miasmatic, chronic nature clearly appeared to me from this circumstance, that after it had once advanced and developed to a
certain degree it can never be removed by the strength of any
robust constitution, it can never be overcome by the most
wholesome diet and order of life, nor will it die out of itself. But it
is evermore aggravated, from year to year, through a transition
into other and more serious symptoms, even till the end of
man's life. . .'

Hahnemann then, believed that chronic diseases remained in
a latent state in the body, returning from time to time in one
form or another. The manifestations may take on the form of an
odinary acute illness, but these were in reality only one event in
a series; and these diseases could only be cured by a remedy
which covered the whole original disease. For example, an
attack of asthma may look like an isolated event in a patient's
history, but on enquiry it will probably be found that the
patient has at some earlier time suffered from a skin eruption.
The asthma and the eruption are both symptoms of the same
disease.

This conclusion was reached by Hahnemann after nearly
twelve years of intensive study and research. For him there were
three sources of chronic infection — Miasms as he called them
— Psora and the two venereal disease Syphilis and Gonorrhoea
which he called Sycosis.

Psora had for its keynote, at some period of the patients

history, an itch-like eruption. In the case of Syphilis a sequence of disease manifestations was known to exist and it has since been proved conclusively that Gonorrhoea similarly attacks the whole constitution producing a chronic sequence of disease manifestations.

The three chronic miasms of Hahnemann were then:

Psora: Contracted or inherited constitutional disease having a non-venereal basis.

Syphilis: The constitutional effects of contracted or inherited syphilis.

Sycosis: The constitutional effects of contracted or inherited gonorrhoea.

Of Psora, Hahnemann writes: 'I had come thus far in my investigations and observations with such non-venereal patients when I discovered . . . that the obstacle of the cure of many cases . . . seemed very often to lie in a former eruption of itch, which was not infrequently confessed; and the beginning of all the subsequent sufferings usually dated from that time. So also with similar chronic patients who did not confess such an infection, or what was probably more frequent, who had, from inattention, not perceived it or, at least, could not remember it. After a careful inquiry it usually turned out that little traces of it (small pustules of itch, herpes, etc.) had showed themselves with them from time to time, even if but rarely, as an indubitable sign of a former infection of this kind.'

'These circumstances, in connection with the fact that innumerable observations of physicians, and not infrequently my own experience, had shown that an eruption of itch suppressed by faulty practice or one which had disappeared from the skin through other means was evidently followed, in persons otherwise healthy by the same or similar symptoms; these circumstances, I repeat, could leave no doubt in my mind as to the internal foe which I had to combat in my medical treatment of such cases.'

He goes on to describe many ailments known to us by their pathological names which have their origin in Psora — skin eruptions, growths, malformations, blood diseases, convulsions, heart-diseases and many others.

He stresses that where eruptions on the skin are suppressed by any means, the disease strikes inwards producing dangerous and often fatal complications, and illustrates his argument with many cases. We give below three of these cases in order that you may follow the strength of his argument.

'A man 30 to 40 years of age had been afflicted with the itch a long time before, and it had been driven away by ointments; from which time he had become more and more asthmatic. His respiration became at last, even when not in motion, very short and extremely laboured, emitting at the same time a continuous hissing sound, but attended with only little coughing. He was ordered an injection of one drachm of squills, and to take internally 3 grains of squills. But by mistake he took the drachm of squills internally. He was near losing his life with an indescribable nausea and retching. Soon after this the itch appeared again on his hands, his feet and his whole body in great abundance, and by this means the asthma was at once removed.'

'A student who had been for a long time afflicted with the itch drove it off with an ointment, and instead of this there broke out ulcers on his arms and legs, and glandular swellings in the armpits. These ulcers were finally cured by external applications when he was seized with dyspnoea and then dropsy, and from these he died.'

'Two youths, brothers, drove off the itch by one and the same remedy, but they lost all appetite, a dry cough and a lingering fever set in, they became emaciated and fell into slumbrous stupor so that they would have died if the eruptions had not luckily re-appeared on the skin.'

So we see that the nature of these chronic miasms is always to act in a direction 'from without inward' as can be realized very clearly in syphilis and sycosis from the nature of their contraction. Although not so clearly perceived with psora, the initial affection is always on the skin where it is easily suppressed by local treatment. Thus the same inward direction is again followed.

Having discovered the existence of a chronically operating poison in the essential character of certain diseases, it was necessary for Hahnemann to find deep acting remedies which corresponded in order to obtain complete similarity. These he named anti-psoric, anti-syphilitic and anti-sycotic and they had to be:

1. Remedies which acted in the opposite direction to the chronic disease — from within outward.

2. Remedies of a deep-acting nature, i.e. capable of affecting profoundly the whole organism, both in its metabolic and physiologic processes, the 'acute' remedies acting only in the sensory and functional sphere.

From this we see that the fourth Law of the Direction of Cure becomes an essential part of Homoeopathic medicine and practice.

Read and study Chapter 22 of Roberts' *The Principles & Art of Cure by Homoeopathy*.

Evacuation of the Bowel

Most healthy people have at least one daily movement of the bowels. But where regular evacuation does not take place a condition of constipation may develop which will result in a state of auto-intoxication; the body will be poisoned by the accumulation of effete matter. This condition can rapidly become chronic and give rise to many subsidiary conditions of health.

The common causes of constipation are:

1. Habit.
2. A 'greedy' colon, i.e. one which absorbs water too quickly.
3. Lack of tone or peristaltic action of the colon muscle.
4. Incorrect diet.

In all cases where constipation is a symptom, careful enquiry will elicit whether habit or diet is at fault.

A history of haemorrhoids may be disclosed as these are often complementary to, or a result of, habitual constipation.

In health the normal stool is of dark brown colour, although ocasionally it may be different according to the nature of the food previously eaten; for example, spinach will cause the stool to be dark green. When an excess of cheese or fat has been taken, the digestive organs may be unable to deal with it, and much is passed which produces a whitish stool.

Black or slatey stools are produced when certain drugs are taken in material doses, as for example, iron and bismuth. A tarry blackness is sometimes imparted when bleeding from the stomach occurs.

Yellow stools are produced in diarrhoea, when the bile is passed almost unchanged. Mucus is almost always a sign of irritation or inflammation in the mucous membrane low down in the bowel. Red blood signifies some diseased condition situated near the lower end of the bowel, e.g. piles. When the blood proceeds from a point higher up it is changed by the action of the digestive juices and resembles coffee grounds.

Diarrhoea, or looseness of the bowels is, except in its mildest forms, a most serious condition. It is a symptom of disease in the bowels, or other organs such as the liver, kidneys, lungs or heart, and may be evidence of their dis-function. In such conditions as cholera, dysentry, typhoid, etc., the extent to which diarrhoea is present is a most important guide to the severity of the condition.

Flatulence is indicative of weakness of tone or nervous action in the stomach (if wind is expelled upwards) or in the bowel (if wind is expelled downwards). Flatulent distention of the abdomen in children often indicates the presence of worms.

Urine

Urine is the excretion produced by the kidneys, and consists chiefly of waste substances resulting from the activity of the body. The urine and the perspiration are to a great extent interdependent; thus, if the kidneys are acting vigorously, there is very little perspiration, whilst if there has been much perspiration, as in fevers, the urine is small in amount and highly concentrated. When the kidneys are diseased, the sweat glands of the skin function more freely.

In composition, urine is made up almost entirely of water, only about 4 per cent being solids in solution. Urea is the most important of the solids, but there are also minute quantities of common salt, phosphates and sulphates combined with potassium, sodium, calcium and magnesium.

In health, the urine is of a light colour. In diseases of the kidneys, such as diabetes and chronic Bright's disease, the urine assumes a very pale colour (the same appearance is, of course, produced after a person has drunk large quantities of water). When blood is present the colour may be pinkish or even bright red according to the amount of haemorrhage, and transparency is lost. Deposits of urates in the urine also give a deep tint and the urine appears cloudy. Where there is any involvement of the liver, bile may be passed when the urine takes on a greenish tint.

The amount of urine passed daily is increased in some diseases notably diabetes and chronic Bright's disease. Feverish conditions and heart diseases cause the amount to be less than normal. Complete stoppage may occur for a time in feverish conditions of children, but in an adult such a state is very serious. When the stoppage is due to a blockage of the ureters by stones, or stricture of the urethra, the secretion by the kidneys still continuing, the condition is known as retention. When the stoppage is due to failure of the kidneys to secrete any urine, the condition is known as suppression or anuria.

Healthy urine has a faint ammoniacal smell, but when it begins to decompose the smell greatly increases and becomes unpleasant. In diabetes the urine has an aroma similar to that of new mown hay. If such a symptom is noted a Homoeopathic Physician should be consulted at once.

In healthy urine there is usually a fleecy deposit of mucus secreted by the mucous membrane of the urinary passages. A pink or yellow deposit, that settles as soon a the urine begins to cool which often leaves a stain upon the utensil in which the urine has stood, is due to urates (uric acid). Uric acid itself, when present, falls in very scanty yellow or brownish grains. A white deposit that collects upon the bottom of the utensil after the urine has stood undisturbed for some time may be due to phosphates, pus, or debris from diseased kidneys known as tube-casts.

Many unusual substances taken into or formed in the body are excreted in the urine. Among these various drugs, disease poisons, bacteria and parasites, but these can only be traced by skilled chemists. Important from the diagnostic viewpoint, how- ever, is the presence in the urine of one of the following: 1) Albumen, 2) Blood, 3) Sugar, 4) Pus and Tube-casts, 5) Bile and 6) Acetone.

Albumen: Present in most kidney diseases, weakening of the heart action, during fever, and in severe anaemia.

It should be noted that in young, active persons there is often a slight degree of albuminaria after exercise, but this is quite normal and if a specimen of urine is taken after rest, e.g. first thing in the morning, no albumen is found.

Blood: Found in acute kidney disease, congestion of the kidneys, or when a stone, ulcer or tumour is present in any of the urinary organs.

Sugar: A sign of diabetes mellitus when it is present constantly in the urine. A diet containing much sugar will cause temporary passing of sugar, but this is to be expected and is of no consequence.

Pus and Tube-casts: Indicate inflammation or ulceration somewhere in the urinary passages. Pus alone generally signifies that the bladder is affected. Tube-casts always point to involvement of the kidneys.

Bile: Signifies that the bile ducts are obstructed, and bile is being absorbed into the blood. Usually a degree of jaundice will be noticeable in the person.

Acetone: May appear in cases of diabetes and general acidosis.

The Appetite

In disease the appetite may become quite depraved with cravings for particular substances and repugnance to others. Such cravings and aversions are very important in the evaluation of symptoms from the Homoeopathic point of view.

There are, however, two chief disorders which deserve special mention, viz: 1) An excessive increase in appetite, and 2) Diminution or loss of appetite.

Excessive appetite may be a bad habit, due to habitual overindulgence in food, leadig to obesity and gouty conditions etc. Where this is elicited in the case history, the necessary advice should be given and an attempt made to guide the patient back to a sensible and more restricted diet. It should be made clear to the patient suffering from excess weight, caused by overindulgence at the table, that he is placing an ever increasing strain upon his heart and other organs. Often sciatica pains of great intensity are entirely relieved in obese persons by reduction of excess weight.

Excessive appetite is sometimes a sign of acid dyspepsia and diabetes. With the latter there is often an intense thirst and in spite of the increased intake of food and drink the person becomes progressively more emaciated.

Diminished appetite is usually found in all diseases which cause general weakness, because the activity of the stomach and the secretion of gastric juices are impaired when vitality is low. Where the appetite is completely lost but there is a corresponding increase in thirst, fever is usually indicated.

Thirst

Thirst, like appetite, is instinctive and means that liquid is necessary for the continuance of bodily activity. In the majority of cases continued thirst indicates fever or inflammation but it may be present in other conditions where a considerable amount of fluid has been lost in the body. Such conditions arise in complaints such as diarrhoea, or after a severe loss of blood.

Thirst may be experienced in acid conditions such as dyspepsia, but usually there will be acid eructations from the stomach as well.

A desire for water is also a feature of any condition of great exhaustion.

Should there however, be no apparent cause for great thirst especially if accompanied by increased heat or dryness of the skin, it can be inferred that it arises from internal heat and is consequently a symptom of fever.

ARSENICUM ALBUM

Characteristics

Restlessness. Great and sudden prostration. Intense burning pains better heat. Intense thirst — drinks often but little at a time. Generally worse at midnight. From midnight until 2 a.m.

Mind: Very restless and anxious and wants to change his position frequently. He becomes suddenly exhausted out of all proportion to the disease.

Head: Pains throbbing and burning, chiefly above one eye or at root of nose — these are better by cold applications and walking in cool air.

Nose: Fluent discharge which corrodes wings of nose and burns; nose gets stopped up; worse out of doors, better in warm room.

Mouth: Dry. Thirst for small drinks but often; worse during perspiration. Lips parched, dry, cracked, corroded and burning from fluent coryza.

Throat: Dry, burning, better warm drinks.

Stomach: Very irritable, least food or drink causes distress and pain. Vomiting and stool simultaneous worse after eating and drinking. Worse cold drinks and ice-cream.

Respiratory:	Difficult breathing worse change of weather. Wheezing. Cannot lie down, must sit up to breathe.
Chest:	Cough with frothy expectoration. Burning in chest.
Limbs:	Pale swellings in joints with burning pains better heat.
Modalities:	Worse cold air; worse cold and damp and from cold things and cold applications; worse 12 midnight until 2 a.m. Worse noon until 2 p.m. Worse movement. Better warm air and hot applications; pains better sweating.

The Arsenicum patient hugs the fire and loves warm wraps but he likes his head cold if he has a headache.

No remedy is more restless than Arsenicum. There is restlessness with great weakness whereas the Aconite restlessness in the earlier stages of illness, fevers etc., is not weak.

There is mental restlessness as well as physical, also great anxiety — and fears — fears of death, that it is useless to take medicine, that he is incurable. There is dislike of disorder — fastidious — described by Dr. Hering as 'the gold-headed cane patient'.

Nash says that Arsenicum leads all the remedies for burning sensations especially in acute diseases — 'There is hardly an organ or tissue in the human system where these burnings of Arsenic are not found'. But the burnings of Arsenicum are improved by heat, i.e. hot applications or heat from the fire or room etc., and remember that the burning throat of Arsenicum is relieved by eating and drinking hot things. There is a burning sensation throughout with aggravation at midnight.

Arsenicum is thought of in food poisoning as it affects the alimentary canal from lips to anus.

Lips dry, parched and cracked.

Tongue dry, and red, or red with indented edges — (it can be white as chalk).

Mouth dry or ulcerated.

Indescribable thirst but can take only a little water at once as the stomach is so very irritable — the least food or drink causes pain, distress, vomiting etc., and sometimes vomiting and stool together. Ice-water and ice-cream particularly disagree.

In respiratory — there is acute coryza — fluent discharge which corrodes lips and nose — much burning when lungs are affected.

Patient cannot lie down.

Affects nervous system — great prostration and characteristic restlessness.

Nash says 'Arsenic is not a panacea — it must, like every other remedy be indicated by its similar symptoms or failure is the outcome. Its great keynotes are restlessness, burning, prostration and midnight aggravation'.

Dr. Tyler says 'Arsenic is not only acrid to mentality, eating into rest — hope — security; but all its secretions and discharges are acrid and corrosive. Acrid tears and eye discharges — acrid nasal discharges; acrid leucorrhoea; acrid burning, corrosive discharges from ulcers which constantly extend in circumference rather than in depth. Burning pains relieved by heat. Worse midnight, after midnight and 1 a.m. specially'.

Kent says 'From the time of Hahnemann to the present day this has been one of the polychrests, one of the most frequently indicated medicines, and one of the most extensively used. . . Arsenic affects every part of man; it seems to exaggerate or depress almost all his faculties, to excite or disturb all his functions . . . it has certain prevailing and striking features. Anxiety, restlessness, prostration, burning and cadaveric odours are prominent characteristics. The surface of the body is pale, cold, clammy and sweating and the aspect cadaveric. The Arsenicum patient with this mental state is always freezing, hovers round the fire, cannot get clothing enough to keep warm, a great sufferer from the cold'.

CHAMOMILLA

Characteristics

Oversensitive to pain. Restlessness. Turmoil in temper. Uncivil. Spiteful.

This remedy is very useful for children.

Mind: Bad temper and irritability to a degree; does not know what he wants; a baby asks for a toy and then hurls it away. Restless. Wants to be carried around; adults walk the floor in agony, the pain

	being out of all proportion to the malady. This patient suffers from the ill'effects of bad temper.
Head:	Pains throbbing or bursting, worse when thinking about them, better by heat. Worse 9 p.m. until midnight.
Ears:	Earache which is better by heat.
Face:	Often one cheek red and the other pale (especially in teething children. Neuralgia worse entering warm room. Toothache worse entering a warm room, better by taking cold water into mouth.
Throat:	Dryness with swelling of tonsils. Spasms in throat during anger, cannot swallow solids. Burning heat.
Respiratory:	Cough associated with earache, dentition etc., hard and dry. Worse 9 p.m. until midnight.
Modalities:	Worse cold damp and windy weather. Chamomilla children are worse 9 a.m. Better warm wet weather and warmth.

Patient is usually chilly, cold and sensitive to cold air and strong winds which annoy him and aggravate his condition.

LEDUM

Characteristics
Pains begin in feet and travel upwards. Blackeye. Puncture wounds. Intense coldness.

Eyes:	Black-eye from a blow or contusion. (Note the 200th potency or Ledum 200 should be used for black-eyes as it is specific).
Limbs:	Gouty pains shoot through foot and limbs and in joints but especially in small joints; swollen, hot, pale. Soles painful, can hardly step on them. Pain starting in foot and travelling up to knee. In acute rheumatism joints swollen and hot but not red. Limbs are cold and cannot get warm and are worse when they do get warm. Swellings are pale and the pains are worse at night, and from the heat of the bed. Relief from cold is very marked and sometimes patients put their feet and legs in

cold water to ease the pains. Ledum for puncture wounds such as sticking the garden fork through the foot or a sharp instrument into the hand. It is an excellent remedy too for stings (especially mos- quito stings) and rat bites as these can also be classed as puncture wounds!

Modalities: Worse warmth and warmth of bed. Worse night. Better cold and cold applications.

TEST PAPER No. 4

These questions should be answered only when the student feels confident that the lesson has been mastered. There should be no reference to books as this would defeat the object.

1. State briefly the difference between acute and chronic disease.

2. Name the three chronic miasms.

3. What must be the nature of remedies which can deal successfully with any of the miasms?

4. Name four characteristics of Arsenicum Album.

Lesson 5

THE PSORIC MIASM

The word Psora was used widely in Hahnemann's time for most of the varied skin troubles known since the earliest times, and so he did not coin the word but rather gave it a deeper meaning. We will quote his own words: 'Psora it is, that oldest, most universal, most pernicious and yet that least known of chronic miasmatic disease, which has been deforming and torturing the nations for thousands of years — the oldest history of the oldest nation does not reach its origin.'

Seven eighths of all chronic maladies prevalent, are ascribed by Hahnemann to psora — the itch.

He says: 'It is an internal disease and may exist *with or without* an eruption on the skin . . . psora became, therefore, the common mother of most chronic diseases . . . the eruptions itch and burn.'

It must be clearly understood, therefore, that psora is an internal disease and that the skin eruption is the manifestation of the disease when it is allowed or forced to come to the surface — and this is the only way it can be eradicated.

Dr. Haehl in *The Life of Hahnemann* says 'To Hahnemann psora is the disease or disposition to disease, hereditary from generation to generation for thousands of years and it is the fostering soil for every possible diseased condition. At the same time it is the most infectious of all. Contact with the general external skin is quite sufficient for transference of the disease in contrast with sycosis and syphilis, in which cases a certain amount of friction on the tenderest parts of our bodies, where most nerves are congregated, and where the cuticle is thinnest, is requisite for infection. But everyone is exposed to psora almost under any circumstances.

'Hereditary transmission for thousands of years, has of course, generated an increasing number of the forms of disease, so that their polymorphous symptoms are nowadays almost

42

innumerable. Hahnemann says that psora, breaking out from its latent state, can be observed in the most variable forms imaginable, according to the bodily constitution, the deficiencies of up-bringing, the habits, the mode of occupation and the external conditions of the individual.

An unusually large number of diseases, stated in the pathology of the older school to be definitely self-existing, are simply 'the characteristic, secondary symptoms of the underlying miasmatic malady now coming to light — namely psora, this thousand headed monster so long undiscovered, so pregnant with misery.'

Hahnemann's great principle in the treatment of psora demands that no skin eruption shall be removed by external remedies. For he realised that a skin eruption is not a local disease but a manifestation of an internal disorder — of unhealthiness — in fact it is a sign of psora.

He says: 'If the physician desires to proceed in a conscientious and intelligent manner, no skin eruption whatever its nature, should be removed by external remedies. The human skin cannot without the help of the rest of the living body produce from itself an eruption. It will never become diseased in any way unless the general diseased condition, the abnormal state of the whole organism, compels it. In every case, an improper condition of the whole body, of the inner living organism, is at the root of the trouble and therefore this must first be considered and should be removed by internal medicines which will alter, improve and cure the whole. Thereupon the eruption depending for existence on the internal disease, will cure itself and disappear — often more speedily than by external remedies.'

The remedies which have a pronounced action in combating this miasm are termed 'anti-Psoric' — their favourable action being demonstrated by the appearance of an eruption or discharge after administration.

The following is a list of the chief anti-psoric remedies:

Agaricus	Arsenicum alb.	Bovista
Alumina	Aurum	Calcarea carb.
Ammonium carb.	Baryta carb.	Carbo animalis
Ammonium mur.	Belladonna	Carbo veg.
Anacardium	Boracic acid	Causticum

Clematis
Colocynth
Conium
Digitalis
Dulcamara
Euphorbium
Graphites
Guaicum
Hepar sulph.
Iodine
Kali carb.
Kali nit.

Lycopodium
Magnesium carb.
Magnesium mur.
Manganum
Mezereum
Muriatic acid
Natrum carb.
Natrum mur.
Nitric acid
Petroleum
Phosphorus
Phosphoric acid

Platinum
Rhododendron
Sarsaparilla
Senega
Sepia
Silica
Stannum
Strontium
Sulphur
Sulphuric acid
Zincum

The anti-psoric remedies are selected in the usual way according to the symptoms and given one dose at a time which must be allowed to work in the body until its action ceases — and this may take 30, 40 or even 50 days — but the fundamental rule is:

'To allow the dose of the medicine, which has been carefully selected for its homoeopathic suitability according to the symptoms of the particular case of disease, to have its effect without interruption as long as it is visibly helping on the cure and increasing to an appreciable extent the improvement of the malady.'

Dr. Haehl says: 'Slight ailments and additional symptoms, such as headache, stiff neck, slight diarrhoea, etc., which may occur during the anti-psoric cure, should not induce a patient to have instant recourse to other medicines, as the effect of the anti-psoric may easily be thereby disturbed or opposed. Such symptoms are very often only the consequence of the remedy acting — a 'homoeopathic aggravation' of moderate extent, a sign of the cure beginning which one may hope with tolerable certainty to see achieved.'

Symptoms of Psora

Psora manifests itself in any part of the body and in many ways, but unless combined with one of the other miasms it never causes structural changes, its sphere being functional disturbances. In order to give you a clearer picture of its action we set out below *some* of the indications of this miasm:

Mind: Mental activity, quick, alert, but easily prostrated from exertion, both mental and physical. A consequent dread of exertion. Anxiety — fears of death, that health will fail, of being unable to succeed. Despondency and mental depression. Thoughts vanish while reading or writing. Ill-effects from strong emotions — grief, fear, etc. Restlessness, and often a longing for travel. Alternating states of gaiety and moodiness.

Head: Vertigo, often specks before the eyes, brought on by motion, looking up quickly, rising from sitting or lying. Morning headaches, constantly returning, persistent, frontal usually. Headaches getting worse during day and improving as night approaches. Hair dry, lustreless, tangles easily, breaks and splits easily. Hair falls out after illness. White spots in the hair. Dry eruptions on the scalp with much itching. Migraine headaches from emotional disturbances.

Eyes: Not greatly affected by psora. Functional disturbances only. Intolerance of daylight or sunlight. Spots before the eyes.

Nose: Increased sensitivity of smell. Greatly affected by odours of any kind which produce nausea, headaches, vertigo, etc.

Face: May be pale, sallow, earthy coloured. Lips very red. Skin usually dry, rough and pimply, having an unwashed or unclean appearance. Acne. In fevers, often red, hot and shining.

Mouth: Taste sour, sweet, or bitter. Perversions of taste generally. Thrush and stomatitis. Herpes.

Chest: Dry, teasing, spasmodic coughs. Functional disturbances of the heart. Violent palpitations with beating of the whole body. Band sensations about the chest. Neuralgic pains about the heart.

Stomach: Always hungry, even with a full stomach. Craving for sweets, acids, sour things. Weak, all-gone sensations. Hunger at night. Hunger and all-gone sensation between 10 a.m. and 11 a.m. Greasy foods aggravate although craved. Prefers hot food.

Abdomen: Flatulence, distention, rumbling, worse at night. Flabby muscles. Cannot tolerate pressure. Abdominal symptoms better from heat.

Urine: Involuntary passing of urine when sneezing, coughing, or laughing. Smarting and burning after urinating.

Stool: Diarrhoeas induced by over-eating, anticipation, usually worse early morning. No desire for stool. Stool dry, scanty, hard, and difficult to expel. Alternation between constipation and diarrhoea. Pin-worms.

Skin: Appears unwashed, and no amount of washing seems to improve it. Dry, rough, dirty, or unhealthy looking. Pruritis. Eruptions worse in open air, better at night. Dry scaly, eruptions. Great itching, with little suppuration.

Extremities: Neuralgic pains. Hands and feet dry, hot, with burning sensations in palms and soles.

Modalities: Worse — sunrise to sunset, after eating, heat of room, standing, approach of menses, new moon. Better — lying down and being quiet (this is an outstanding characteristic in most complaints), heat slow movement, weeping, diarrhoeas, perspiration, urinating.

Generals: Functional disturbances. Weak and debilitated persons. Dropsical symptoms. Coldness in most ailments. Easy fatigue. The 'great unwashed'.

Read and study Chapters 23, 24 and 25 of Roberts' *The Principles and Art of Cure by Homoeopathy*

EXPECTORATION

Expectoration varies considerably in character according to the diseases with which it is associated.

An important consideration is the ease with which the sputum is expectorated. Where it is expelled by an effort, such as repeated hawking or coughing, or where there is more or less acute pain or soreness in the effort to detach it, a continued irritation and obstruction of the air-cells and passages is evidenced. On the other hand, when the sputum is discharged with ease, there is no pain, and great relief is experienced, it is an indication that the acute stage of any inflammatory condition of the throat or lungs has passed. The appearance of the expectoration at this time may be of a thick yellowish nature, occasionally modified by a few slight streaks of blood.

At the beginning of inflammatory conditions, such as acute bronchitis or inflammation of the throat, there may be much cough yet little expectoration. The cough is usually painful and dry. During the greater part of an attack of acute bronchitis, particularly in old people, the expectoration is of a watery, frothy character and is brought up in considerable quantities.

Where the sputum appears jelly-like or sticky and is tinged with a 'rusty' colur, a severe inflammation of the lungs is indicated. This type of expectoration is found when the patient is suffering from pneumonia and often the sputum in this disease is so sticky that it adheres to the vessel into which it is expectorated, even when the latter is turned upside down.

Haemoptysis, or bleeding from the lungs, is an extremely serious condition and medical aid must be sought immediately. Usually, it indicates pulmonary tuberculosis or carcinoma of the lung.

It should be borne in mind, however, that spitting of blood may be due merely to a bleeding from the nose when the blood has run into the throat; or to the rupture of a small vessel on the wall of the throat when this part of the air passage is inflamed.

Bleeding from the stomach is different from Haemoptysis as it is usually dark brown and granular in appearance. It should be noted that blood from the stomach is *always vomited* and results generally from some ulcerated or congested state.

Expectoration like 'prune juice' occurring in the course of pneumonia is an ominous sign, and usually indicates that softening of parts of the lungs has begun.

A yellow, bitter-tasting expectoration indicates an affection of the liver.

THE TONGUE

Many of the most important indications associated with derangement of the digestive functions can be observed from the state of the tongue. In health the surface of the tongue should be smooth with a slight groove in the middle. The edge of the tongue should be sharp and even. It is under the control of the will and can be moved in any direction.

Where the tongue is flabby, large and pale, and shows teeth marks along its edge, a condition of general debility in the muscular system is indicated.

Tremulousness when the tongue is protruded is indicative of

a nervous condition usually found in persons who indulge too heavily in alcoholic drinks; a symptom of considerable importance, as it may be the only sign of this weakness.

Dryness of the tongue points to diminished secretion, and is common in acute and inflammatory diseases.

In eruptive fevers a very red tongue is often observed. In gastric and bilious fevers, and in severe indigestion, the redness may be limited to the edges and tip.

In scarlet fever there is often seen what is called a 'Strawberry Tongue', the general surface being covered with a white fur, through which project the red and inflamed points of the larger papillae with which the tongue is studded.

Thickly furred, dirty white, and possibly slimy indicates derangement of the lining membrane of the stomach. Where the fur is of a yellowish colour, the liver is also possibly involved.

Where the tongue shows white patches interspersed with sharply marked red, bare areas, the condition is known as a mapped or 'geographical tongue'. It is a mild form of inflammation in which the surface layer of the mucous membrane on the tongue peels off, and it is usually associated with digestive disorders and a degree of general debility.

In all complaints the gradual cleaning of the tongue, first from the tip and edges, shows a tendency to health and indicates a general cleansing of the whole alimentary tract.

SULPHUR

Sulphur is one of the greatest 'polychrests' (drugs of many uses) and is Hahnemann's Prince of 'antipsorics'. Hahnemann says of Sulphur: 'The homoeopathic physician (who alone acts in conformity with natural laws) will meet many important morbid states for which he will discover and may expect much asistance in the symptoms of Sulphur and Hepar Sulphuris'.

Kent says 'Sulphur is such a full remedy that it is somewhat difficult to tell where to begin. It seems to contain a likeness of all the sicknesses of man, and a beginner on reading over the proving of Sulphur might naturally think that he would need no other remedy, as the image of all sickness seems to be contained in it.

'The Sulphur patient is a lean, lank, hungry, dyspeptic fellow with stoop shoulders, yet many times it must be given to fat, rotund, well-fed people. The angular, lean, stoop-shouldered patient, however, is the typical one, and especially when he has become so from long periods of indigestion, bad assimilation and feeble nutrition. The Sulphur state is sometimes brought about by being long housed up and adapting the diet to the stomach. Persons who lead sedentary lives, confined to their rooms in study, in meditation, in philosophical inquiry, and who take no exercise, soon find out that they must eat only the simplest of foods, foods not sufficient to nourish the body, and they end up by going into a philosophical mania . . . another class of patients in whom we see a Sulphur appearance in the face; dirty, shrivelled, red-faced people. If it be a child, the mother may wash the face often, but it always looks as if it had been perfunctorily washed. The Sulphur scholar, the inventor, works day and night in threadbare clothes and battered hat; he has long, uncut hair and a dirty face; his study is uncleanly, it is untidy; books are piled up indiscriminately; there is no order. It seems that Sulphur produces this state of disorder . . . uncleanliness, a state of 'don't care how things go,' and a state of selfishness. He becomes a false philosopher . . . disappointed because the world does not consider him the greatest man on earth . . . he has on a shirt that he has worn many weeks; if he has not a wife to attend to him, he would wear his shirt until it fell from him'.

Nash says: 'No remedy has more general, positive and persistent action upon the skin than Sulphur. With or without eruption, itching and burning are the characteristic sensations attending the skin symptoms. If any one doubts the itch-producing power of Sulphur, let him work a day or two in the bleaching room of a broom factory. I have tried this experiment and we all remember the fact that our mothers and grandmothers used to cure or rather over-cure itch with it. So strong is the affinity of Sulphur for the skin that it seems bent on pushing everything internal out on the surface. Especially is this true if it is something that naturally belongs there.'

The full use of Sulphur can only be appreciated when one realizes the true implications of Psora but one must also remember that Sulphur is not the only anti-psoric remedy.

However, as Nash says 'it may be as well to speak of the power possessed by Sulphur of arousing or exciting defective reaction. Your former remedy was well chosen and seemed to help in a measure, but the case relapses, lingers or progresses slowly to perfect recovery. It is on account of a depression of the vital force, as Hahnemann would call it. It may be on account of psora or not. Now give a dose of Sulphur and let it act for a few hours if in an acute case, or a number of days if chronic. Then you may return to your former remedy and get results which you could not before the Sulphur was given. It clears up the case and prevents its becoming chronic or a lingering unsatisfactory convalescence.'

Characteristics

Extremely red orifices, especially lips as if painted red. Empty, gone, faint, hungry sense at pit of stomach around 11 a.m. must have something to eat or drink. Offensive odour of body despite frequent washing. Aversion to bathing; it aggravates. Burning heat on top of head, of palms, and especially of soles of feet at night in bed, must put feet out of bed to cool them off. Worse standing. Fluids all burn parts over which they pass.

Mind:	Easily angered; fault finding; irritable; restless and quarrelsome. Foolish happiness and pride, thinks he has the best of everything. Hates to either work or be washed. Always theorising. Wants to know the why and wherefore of everything. Dwells on useless speculation.
Head:	Headache every Sunday.
Eyes:	Lids very red.
Ears:	Very red.
Mouth:	Lips very red.
Stomach:	Worse 11 a.m. (Sinking, all gone faint hungry feeling.) Craves sweets.
Anus:	Very red.
Skin:	Itching better scratching and then it burns.
Modalities:	Worse standing: worse 11 a.m. in a close room; open air; bathing; cold damp weather. Better doors and windows open: sitting or lying.

Sulphur, Calcarea and Lycopodium are the trio of remedies on which the whole of the Materia Medica is based.

If you have a patient suffering from any named ailment and he exhibits three or more of the *characteristics* of sulphur, then you can prescribe it with confidence — i.e. burning, redness, itching, offensive odours, unkempt and unclean, worse 11 a.m. and worse standing.

CALCAREA CARBONICA

This is the trituration of the middle layer of the oyster shell.

The sweats are general — night sweats and on exertion especially on head, neck and chest — this often applies to children.

The skin is white, watery or chalky, pale — and the disposition torpid and sluggish or slow in movement.

Sulphur Calcarea, and Lycopodium are a trio of remedies that should be studied and compared. Note the sluggish or slow movements of Calc. carb. and the almost opposite quick, wiry nervous active movements of Sulphur; then again there is none of the bilious swarthy yellowish appearance in Calc. carb. that we find in Lycopodium.

From Hering's 'Guiding Symptoms' we quote 'Tardy development of the bony tissues with lymphatic enlargements. Curvature of the bones especially spine and long bones. Extremities deformed, crooked. Softening of the bones, fontanels remain open too long, and skull very large.'

Nash says that Calcarea shows the lack of or imperfect nutrition of bones. Whilst they are not nourished evenly or properly the soft parts are suffering from over nutrition and thus we get soft flabby people especially in children and young people.

The sensation of coldness is a characteristic of Calcarea — the opposite to the burning of Sulphur. There are partial sweats — in all sweatings of Calcarea the surface of the skin is characteristically cold.

The digestive tract is sour — there are sour eructations sour vomiting, sour diarrhoea, sour mucus and sour smell of whole body. The diarrhoea is worse in the afternoon. The patient is usually better when constipated.

Dr. Tyler says 'The fat, flabby child is brought in and dumped down on to a chair and sits there. No wriggling down to wander about and touch everything in the room. She sits there, lethargic and dull. Perhaps plays with her fingers and picks them. With the chalky complexion goes — fatness without fitness — sweating without heat — bones without strength and tissue of plus quantity and minus quality. More flabby bulk with weariness and weakness. In Calc. everything is slow and late and heavy and weak'.

Kent says that Calc children have dreadful times in their dreams and in an adult you can often recognise Calcarea by the limp, cold moist handshake.

FEARS — that something is going to happen to herself or somebody else — that she will lose her reason, and people will notice — that people will notice her confusion of mind. Fearfulness with restlessness and vague fears — fears of death. Broods over little things of no importance — peevish, fretful — obstinate. Calcarea is a very tired patient.

Kent says 'It is a peculiar feature of Calcarea that the more marked the congestion of internal parts, the colder the surface becomes. With chest troubles, the stomach troubles, and bowel troubles, the feet and hands become like ice, and covered with sweat; and he lies in bed sometimes with a fever in the rest of the body, and the scalp covered with cold sweat. That is strange. You cannot account for that by any reasoning in pathology, and when a thing is so strange that it cannot be accounted for, it becomes very valuable as descriptive of the remedy, and is one that cannot help but be of value when prescribing for the patient.'

The headaches begin in occiput and spread to top of head and are so severe that they feel as if they will burst.

Calcarea is the chronic of Belladonna — i.e. when Belladonna has again and again helped the acute condition Calcarea will be curative and so prevent its recurrence.

Characteristics

Coldness, general and local, subjective and objective. Sweats, especially about head, feet and hands. Head covered with cold sweat when other parts of body are comfortable. Sweats even in cold room and in cold air. Sweats on face when nowhere else. Feet sweat on becoming very cold or very warm. Fearful. Sensitive to cold and damp weather but patients cannot sit in the sun. Feels as though he has on damp stockings.

Mind: Very fearful and apprehensive — FULL OF FEARS. Melancholy. Depressed. Mentally and physically always tired.

Head: Profuse cold sweat (often to be found in babies and pillow is soaked.) Sweat from least exertion. Pain as if in vice. Congestion of head.

Face: Chalky, white, bloodless.

Mouth: Unpleasant taste mostly sour. Sour risings. Desires strange food, limes, slate pencils, eggs, earth, chalk, clay, raw potatoes, sweets, ice-cream.

Stomach: Sinking empty sensation at any time. Vomit sour.

Respiratory: Breathless worse ascending. Cough with expectoration of thick, grey mucus — sour.

Chest: Congestion. Shortness of breath. Oppression of chest. Anxious feeling in chest.

Neck and Back: Glands under the lower jaw tender, worse moving jaw; worse touch.

Limbs: Pain in joints worse on becoming cold; worse cold wet weather; worse cold wind. Numbness of legs worse evening. Cramps worse 3 a.m. Stiffness worse night. Feet and legs cold and clammy (sensation as if in damp stockings). Hands cold and clammy — (handshake feels boneless, moist and cold).

Modalities: Worse cold; cold damp; worse change of weather especially to damp, it goes right through them; worse draughts, from working in water and bathing; worse full moon; after midnight and early morning; on awakening.

These patients are very chilly and dread the open air; they are sensitive to cold damp air and to draughts. They catch cold very easily.

TEST PAPER No. 5

These questions should be answered only when the student feels confident that the lesson has been mastered. There should be no reference to books as this would defeat the object.

1. How would you expect a psoric disease to respond to Homoeopathic treatment?

2. If a patient complained of a skin eruption what advice would you give him and what other conditions would you expect to find?

3. Describe an imaginary child who would respond, in your opinion, to a dose of Sulphur.

Lesson 6

THE SYPHILITIC MIASM

Syphilis is a comparatively modern disease, but is the basis of many constitutional troubles. Let us first consider the contraction of the disease and its effects on the body. In Hahnemann's words — 'In impure coition the specific infection probably takes place instantaneously at the point of contact and friction.

'When the infection has taken hold, the whole living body is overcome with it. Directly after the moment of infection the formation of venereal disease begins in the whole of the interior . . . It is only after this penetration of the evil received into all the organs, only when the transformation of the whole man into a venereal subject . . . is complete . . . that the morbid state tries to ease and to palliate the internal evil by producing a local symptom (called a chancre) which first appears as a blister and then breaks out into a painful sore.'

We are not concerned in the primary contraction of syphilis. But we *are* concerned with the *effects* of the disease which have filtered down through generations affecting the constitutions of the children.

What are these effects? Syphilis is a deadly poison once driven internally, eating into the system, destroying certain constituent elements in tissues and altering the structure of bones and ligaments. In the first generation the off-spring of parents suffering from the disease show deep constitutional faults such as deformities and malformations, chronic catarrhal conditions, ulcers etc. The primary symptoms of the disease are not so apparent in the off-spring, the internal organs of the parents having already been contaminated by the disease.

In the second, and succeeding generations, these various manifestations gradually lose their major proportions and a tendency towards normality is observed. That this corrective process is a natural law can be demonstrated in other forms of life. For instance, artificially produced strains of flowers always tend to 'throw-back' to their natural form, and it is a comforting thought that even the deadliest of man's diseases will tend to die out over the course of time, providing no other miasm has been introduced. It should be realised that rarely is one miasm alone active in a person, each of us inheriting the constitutional faults of both paternal and maternal ancestors.

In order to obtain a composite picture of the effects of syphilis, let us study some of the manifestations.

The chief characteristics are:

1. Deformed or altered construction
2. Indurations and ulcerations, and
3. A nightly aggravation of all complaints.

Mind: The person is slow of comprehension, sullen, stupid, easily angered, suspicious. Dread of the night. Obstinacy. Keeps his troubles to himself. Gets fixed ideas which no amount of reasoning wil remove. Mental troubles relieved by the breaking out of an ulcer, haemorrhage. Extreme types — criminals, sadists.

Head: Dull and heavy headaches, usually commencing at the base of the head. These are sometimes one-sided, always worse at night, and getting better as morning approaches. Large heads, with profuse perspiration, giving off an unpleasant odour. Moist eruptions with yellow pus. Hair falls out in handfuls leaving bare spots, commencing at the vertex. Matted hair, smelling badly.

Eyes: Malformation of eyeball. Ulcerations and inflammations. Dread of artificial light.

Ears: Abscesses. Discharges from the ear. Meningeal troubles.

Nose: Snuffles. Ulceration. Dark, greenish, black or brown crusts. Destruction of nasal bones.

Face: Greyish, greasy appearance. Deep fissures in the lips. Children look old puckered, dried up, like old men.

Mouth: Ulcers. Deformed teeth, decaying early. Upper and lower jaw out of alignment.

Stomach: Aversion to meat. Desires cold food and drink.

	Many disturbances caused by too rich a diet.
Chest:	Changes in the structure of the chest.
Abdomen:	Sudden and severe diarrhoeas.
Skin:	Eruptions about joints, flexures of the body, and arranged in circular groupings. Copper coloured or raw-ham colour. Thick and heavy scales. Varicose ulcers are the last destructive manifestations on the skin. Ecchymoses and haemorrhagic conditions.
Generals:	Destruction of tissue. The periosteum and long bones especially attacked. Growing pains in children. All complaints worse at night and at the approach of storms.

Hahnemann gave one remedy as being absolutely curative of uncomplicated Syphilis — Mercury. He emphasized that it should be 'the smallest dose of the best mercurial preparation.' Such symptoms as we shall observe, however, will be altered in character as we are endeavouring to recognise the *inherited* taint only. Many remedies may therefore be indicated according to the constitutional background of each individual, but these remedies will fall into the group of deep-acting remedies as Calc. fluor., Aurum., Acid fluor., Kali bich., etc.

Read and study Chapters 26, 27 and 28 of Roberts' *The Principles and Art of Cure by Homoeopathy*

The Sycotic Miasm

Sycosis, the 'fig-wart' disease, is the after effects of suppressed gonorrhoeal poison. When gonorrhoea has been naturally treated and thoroughly and completely cured, sycosis rarely develops. When, however, gonorrhoea has been suppressed and its poisons driven back into the system, the full destructive nature of the disease becomes apparent.

The first symptoms after suppression usually appear in anaemia and inflammatory conditions of any part of the body. Later symptoms take on many forms, but sycotic manifestations generally tend to infiltration and over-growth of tissue — warts and warty growths, deposits in the joints and tissues leading to rheumatic complaints, thickening of the skin and nails. The pelvic and sexual organs especially are attacked by this miasm.

This sycotic poison can be handed on. It is, however, not transmitted in its original form; the symptoms passed on are those which are manifest at the time of the transmission. Where, for example, a healthy woman marries a man who has suffered from gonorrhoea, which has been supposedly 'cured', it has been found that the woman's health begins to deteriorate and secondary symptoms begin to appear similar to those mentioned above. Children born to such a union inherit the taint, and again show similar symptoms. Thus the suppressed gonorrhoeal poison is handed down from father to son. In many patients, traces of the inherited disease may be observed, and these can only be eradicated by correctly chosen anti-sycotic remedies.

It has also been observed that when a person has been vaccinated repeatedly similar symptoms manifest themselves. It is interesting to note that the manner of infection is similar to that of the miasms, viz: Infection takes place the moment the vaccine enters the blood stream. Then follows the period during which the whole organism is infected, when there is a more or less vigorous reaction and an attempt by the vital force to throw the poison out at the place of entry. Then the struggle ceases and the body accommodates itself to the intruder. In re-vaccination the body often has no further resistance to offer but suffers the additional weight of poison material silently and it is assumed that the vaccination 'did not take'! Yet later, symptoms begin to appear similar in character to the true sycotic poison, and only by skilful treatment can this destructive tendency be halted, and the sick person brought back to health.

In modern times, therefore, sycosis has taken on a double meaning, i.e. the morbid conditions develop as a result of:

1. Inherited gonorrhoeal poison, or
2. Repeated vaccination.

Hahnemann's remedies for sycosis were Thuja and Nitric Acid. He states: 'Both the gonorrhoea and the excrescences of sycosis are cured in the most durable way by the internal administration of a few globules of Thuja, which should be allowed to act for 15, 20, 30 or 40 days. After this you may give an equally small dose of Nitric Acid, letting it act for a like period. These two remedies are sufficient to cure both the sycosis and the excrescences. In inveterate cases the larger excrescences may be touched once a day with the fresh juice of Thuja, diluted with equal parts of alcohol.'

As in syphilis, however, in the treatment of *inherited* sycosis, many remedies may be indicated and the prescription must be based on the totality of the symptoms. Where this disease is recognised it is, nevertheless, often found of great value to give a dose of Thuja 200 in order to 'clear the way' for the indicated remedy.

Some of the chief indications of the sycotic miasm are as follows:

Mind:	Cross, irritable. Worse when the weather changes. Fixed ideas. Jealousy and suspicion. Forgets recent events, but remembers old events quite clearly. Self condemnation. Suicidal. Degenerates. All mental conditions better on reappearance of a discharge or other elimination.
Head:	Headaches at vertex or frontal. Worse at or after midnight. Headache always better from motion. Vertigo at base of the brain. Hair falls out in circular spots.
Nose:	Red and studded with capillaries. Sense of smell lost. Discharge with odour of fish-brine. Snuffles in children. Yellowish green catarrh. Cannot breathe through the nose owing to accumulation of mucus.
Mouth:	Musty or fishy taste.
Face:	Congested, blue. Warty eruptions. Hair of beard falls out.
Chest:	Violent hammering of the heart with other complaints. Heart pains better by gentle exercise. Pain from shoulder to heart with rheumatic conditions.
Stomach:	Worse after eating, pain relieved by lying on stomach. Crampy or colicky pains, better from hard pressure. Fond of beer, rich foods, fat meats, highly seasoned foods.
Abdomen:	Pains better hard pressure, bending double. Colic. Appendicitis and peritonitis.
Female:	Ovarian inflammation, uterine disorders, cysts. Catarrhal discharges, yellowish-green, with fish-brine odour. Colic with menses. Leucorrhoea

	thin, scanty, acrid, producing biting or itching and burning of the parts.

Stool: Fluent, forceful diarrhoea preceded by colic. Acid, corrosive.

Skin: Warts and warty growths. Moles. Wine coloured patches. Nails ribbed, ridged, thick, and heavy. Barbers itch.

Extremities: Rheumatic conditions. Tearing in joints, worse during rest, cold damp weather. Better moving or stretching and in dry weather. Pain in small joints with infiltration and deposits. Pains worse at approach of storm.

Generals: Inflammatory rheumatism of soft tissues. Slowness of recovery. General relief by discharges. Pains alternate with discharges. Neuralgias. Fish-brine odour of all discharges. Greenish or greenish-yellow discharges. Susceptibility to rheumatic conditions. Arthritis deformans, with deposits of lime salts.

Illustration of Sycotic Miasm

This brings to mind the patient who came for treatment with gout. After eating the smallest portion of meat the big toe on the left foot would become inflamed and extremely painful — it would wear off in two or three days if no more meat was taken.

On taking the totality of the symptoms it was found that Urtica Urens was needed and although three doses in the 30th potency were given, her condition was improved but not cured.

On careful consideration it was realised that gout is a disease that is nearly always traced back to the sycotic miasm and a unit dose of Medorrhinum 200 was given as it was revealed that as a child she had chronic catarrh (which she had 'grown out of') and also she had a wart on her cheek.

After a week her symptoms still called for Urtica Urens and this was then given — one dose in the 200th potency. This was six years ago and although this woman now eats meat in normal quantities she has never had a return of gout.

The remedy medorrhinum used in this case is known as a 'nosode'.

Read and study Chapters 29 and 30 of Roberts' *The Principles and Art of Cure by Homoeopathy.*

PAIN

Among the many symptoms of disease, the symptoms of pain are perhaps the most frequently complained about. The student will have learnt in previous lessons, that it is on the *totality* of symptoms that a Homoeopathic remedy is prescribed, and *not* on any one particular affection or indication of disease; nevertheless the repeated complaints of sick people in regard to their aches and pains cannot and must not be entirely disregarded and we are therefore devoting some time to a closer examination of this distress signal, for such it most certainly is. Pain is always an indication of some greater disharmony and care should be taken to record its exact nature.

Pain is a single symptom. It is not a reliable guide to a remedy but must be taken into consideration with other symptoms to be of value. It must be borne in mind that we have no way of measuring pain but must estimate the patient's tolerance of it. This is often referred to as the patient's 'threshold' of discomfort. What is severe pain to a sensitive, nervous, or exhausted person, might be mere discomfort to one who is habitually phlegmatic, or in robust health.

Generally pain is described in various ways by each patient, but it is helpful to remember that the sensation produced in the majority of persons in various conditions comes under several main groupings as follows:

Throbbing: Usually indicates an inflammatory condition, and where the affection is serious the pain may be severe. Inflammation usually produces an uninterrupted pain in a localised area and is worse by pressure.

Boring: Often indicates pressure, ulceration or inflammatory conditions. Where bone is affected the pain may be excruciating in character.

Gnawing: The pain of a stomach ulcer is often described in this way but the expression is usually found in association with the growth of tumours and great care should be taken where this symptom is given.

Aching, bruised, stiff: This may be simply the after-effect of the over-use of a muscle. In well established cases of stiffness with aching actual deposits in the tissues of fatigue products may be present. Rheumatism deposits cause similar symptoms usually localising in a particular joint or muscle.

Griping, colicky: Irritation of such organs as the bowels, bile-ducts, bladder or ureters will cause this type of pain, the patient usually being compelled to double up in order to obtain relief.

Burning: Often descriptive of dyspeptic pains caused by an excess of acid in the gastric juices irritating the nerve endings in the stomach membrane.

Shooting: Usually indicates that pain is travelling along the course of a nerve. It can, therefore, be assumed that there is some irritation of a nerve in the stated area.

The above definitions are necessarily brief and one must learn to interpret the statement of the patient in his description of the pain which he is suffering. Inflammation usually causes a pain which is continuous in a specified area and is worse by pressure. Where pain runs in a particular direction and appears worse from slight touch, but is ameliorated from heavy pressure, it is nervous in character. Pain which comes and goes in the same part or parts and is cramp-like or constrictive in character, relieved by warmth or pressure, indicates spasm of the part affected.

Observation of the part is often of assistance in confirming the nature of the pain. For instance, where the pain is caused by inflammation there will be increased heat of the whole body — fever, high pulse rate and severe thirst. Nervous pains are always of an irregular nature — darting, dragging, pulsating, shooting — and there may be an increase of heat along the course of the affected nerve. But the person will be holding the part tightly, or sitting in such a way as to exert pressure on the nerve. Spasmodic pains such as colic, cause the person to double up by the severity of the contraction — but feverish symptoms will be unlikely.

Remember, however, our opening remarks on the nature of pain. Always pay close attention to the complementary symptoms before deciding on the type of pain presented in any case.

THE PULSE

Pulse readings provide a quick estimate of the general condition of the patient and the state of his circulation, i.e. if strong, full and hard an inflammatory condition is present.

The term 'The pulse' refers to the pulse wave of the radial artery which, because of its superficial position and easy accessibility is the one usually felt with the fingers. The wave is not a forward movement of a column of blood but is actually an advancing wave produced by blood being ejected into the aorta independent of the speed of the blood flow.

Reading the Pulse:

The patient should be at ease both mentally and physically. Anything which tends to excite the action of the patient's heart defeats the object in view.

Three fingers are placed upon the radial artery (inner side of the wrist) with the thumb on the opposite side. A variation in the degree of pressure will indicate the *nature* of the beats, i.e. soft, full, hard. The *number* of beats per minute are carefully counted.

Normal Pulse:

The healthy pulse is uniform, equal, moderately full, and swelling slowly under the fingers. It is smaller and quicker in women and children and in old age the pulse becomes hard owing to increased firmness or to structural change in the arterial coats.

The average number of beats per minute are as follows:

Birth 140	Infancy 120—130	Childhood 100
Youth 90	Adults 75	Old age 65—70
	Senility 75—80	

These readings are for the average person. Various circumstances will affect the readings considerably, viz: after exercise or excitement the pulse is quicker. The readings are faster when the person is standing rather than sitting and faster sitting than lying. As a result of cold, sleep, fatigue or want of food the readings will be slower.

Regular pulse readings in acute cases help to determine the degree of progress made by the disease upon the vital force, and consequently the seriousness of the illness is more easily assessed.

A number of varying titles have been given to the characteristics observed in reading the pulse, the following being those generally in use:

Full: Occurs in plethoric conditions or in the early stages of acute diseases.

Weak: Feeble conditions of the system.

Rapid: If strong, full and hard it indicates inflammation or fever. If small and very rapid it points to a stage of great debility.

Jerking: A quick rather forcible beat, followed by a sudden, abrupt cessation, as if the direction of the wave of blood has been reversed. Heart disease is usually indicated.

Intermittent: A pulsation is occasionally omitted, frequently owing to some obstruction in the circulation in the heart and lungs. It may also be observed in some forms of valvular diseases of the heart and in apoplexy. Prolonged over-exertion, anxiety, or flatulence may produce it. Often a symptom of a gouty constitution.

Note: In acute diseases an unequal or changeable pulse denotes the complaint as nervous in origin and *not* inflammatory. Thus although the pains complained of, even throbbing, may seem to indicate inflammation, if the pulse is unequal the trouble may be spasmodic or neuralgic.

THUJA

This remedy is Hahnemann's chief anti-sycotic, and it is given to patients who frequently say 'I have never been well since vaccination'.

Modalities — worse cold, damp air, after vaccination, excessive tea drinking, extension of limbs; better drawing up limbs.

The mental symptoms are curious — patient thinks that the body and particularly the limbs are made of glass and will readily break. When walking he feels as though his legs are made of wood. He feels as though a living animal were in the abdomen. Full of fixed ideas. Makes mistakes in speaking and writing — speaks slowly and has prolonged thoughfulness about the merest trifles.

There is a great deal of croaking, rumbling and grumbling in abdomen as of an animal crying. The abdomen is puffed and big.

Chronic constipation with hard, black large stools, or diarrhoea — forcibly expelled, copious gurgling like water from a bung hole of a barrel — diarrhoea especially from effects of vaccination.

One of its black letter symptoms is 'on exposure of the body to warm air, shivering all over'. Rigor with much yawning, the warm air feels cold to him and the sun seems to have no power of warmth.

Thuja's warts are soft, pulpy and very sensitive; they burn, itch and bleed easily when rubbed by clothing.

Dr. Clarke says of Thuja 'People are all vaccinated and drink tea and Thuja is the great antidote to tea and vaccination'.

Dr. Tyler says 'And now a word of warning to homoeopaths in regard to Thuja. It is not a safe drug in careless or ignorant hands. The 'Thuja-disease where the remedy is persisted in, may also become chronic, according to Kent. We will quote. . .' 'If you repeat again and again, you will have that which will remain a life-time. . . Crude drugs do not impress the vital force so lastingly; but an individual who is thoroughly sensitive . . . as sensitive as contagion, then if you undertake to prove (in potency) by giving it night and morning, you will rivet upon him a lifelong miasm'.

Always the greater the power the greater its capabilities for good and evil and the more the knowledge needed for its employment. And I think we have proved that Thuja is, as Hahnemann says 'an uncommonly powerful medicinal substance . . . useful in some of the most serious diseases of mankind, for which hitherto there has been no remedy.'

MERCURIUS

Characteristics:
Aching, especially in bones and where flesh is thin over the bones. Swollen, flabby tongue taking imprint of teeth. Gums swollen, spongy, bleeding. Breath very offensive. Sweats day and night without relief in many ailments. Moist tongue (saliva) with intense thirst. Creeping chilliness at beginning of cold.

Mind:	Restless 8 p.m. Time seems to pass slowly.
Nose:	Discharge or catarrh thin and excoriating, becoming thicker, greenish and more bland. Coryza better on becoming heated.
Mouth:	Gums spongy, sometimes bleeding; tongue swollen, flabby and taking imprint of teeth. Whole mouth moist with saliva, the odour very offensive. Intense thirst.
Throat:	Tonsils greatly swollen.
Limbs:	Sharp and lancinating pains in hip joints, thighs and knees worse evening and night and during movement and often with a sensation of coldness in diseased parts.
Modalities:	Worse by heat and worse by cold. Worse at night.

Patients needing this remedy are human barometers and every change of temperature worsens their condition.

TEST PAPER No. 6

These questions should be answered only when the student feels confident that the lesson has been mastered. There should be no reference to books as this would defeat the object.

1. List six manifestations that would lead you to suspect that the Syphilitic Miasm was present.

2. Give six indications that would point to Sycosis being present.

3. With regard to the Sycotic Miasm, what else must be taken into account, in addition to inherited gonorrhoeal poison?

4. Thuja is a great antidote to:

   a) ....

   b) ....

Lesson 7

COMBINED MIASMS

We stated earlier that rarely will one observe in any patient the uncomplicated effect of one miasm. We are born with our inheritance of Psora in greater or lesser degree on to which may be grafted either or both of the other miasms. The truly chronic case, therefore, presents a multiplicity of symptoms and it is our task to recognise the underlying cause and to eliminate the taints if possible by attacking them with the correctly indicated remedy.

We must, then, be able to recognise the traces of the underlying causes, however faint, before we can do good work. Let us briefly sum up what we have learned from our study so far of the miasms.

Psora: This is the oldest. Its main sphere of action is on the skin, where, if undisturbed it forms a pruritis followed by a finer vesicular eruption. Suppressive treatment changes its character and drives it inward to the vital organs setting up functional derangements, an alteration in metabolism, and hence deficiency diseases and weakness from malnutrition.

Altered metabolism is evident in the psoric patient by his constant desire to eat even after a meal, leading to over-strain of the digestive organs and consequent troubles in the digestive system.

The weakness from malnutrition is further evidenced by the constant desire to lie down and rest.

The skin of the psoric patient is dirty and unhealthy and there is often an intense skin irritation. He looks unclean in himself and in his clothes, and his hair is always untidy and will not stay in place.

Mentally he is timid and anxious. He is quick and active, but easily prostrated with mental exhaustion. Any emotional disturbance will upset him and make him ill.

Sycosis: The miasm resulting from suppressed gonorrhoea. Its action is to attack the blood producing an anaemia, involving under-nourishment and deterioration of every cell in the body. This anaemic condition can be observed in the pale, ashy grey colour of the face. The nose is often red with prominent capillaries.

Sycosis infiltrates into the tissues causing catarrhs, fibroid growths, tumours and warts. The discharges are characterised by their offensive fish-brine odour. This miasm selects the pelvic organs for many of its manifestations and ailments such as menstrual disorders, growths in the uterus, leucorrhoea and troubles of child-bearing evidence its presence in the organism.

Mentally the sycotic patient is irritable, jealous and suspicious. All his troubles are worse in the cold, damp weather.

Syphilis: This manifests itself in ulceration and destruction of tissue. Soft tissue such as is found in the mouth, nose and throat, is especially susceptible to its action. The long bones and periosteum are also attacked. The teeth are deformed and the upper and lower jaw are out of alignment. There are also bodily deformities of all kinds. Mentally the patient with the syphilitic background is sulky, morose, stubborn, depressed, stupid and slow in comprehension. Worse at night and at the approach of storms are two strong modalities.

Having the general action of the miasms firmly in mind we can now proceed to consider their effects when combined in a patient. We see that the combinations can be as follows:

1. Psora combined with syphilis.
2. Psora combined with sycosis.
3. Psora combined with syphilis and sycosis.

Psora and Syphilis: This combination presents us with the picture of the tubercular constitution and shows itself in various forms such as lung phthisis, scrofula, etc., and also in acute forms such as meningitis.

Brief notes on the tubercular constitution have been given in Lesson 3 but in order to recognise this combination we give below a more detailed description.

The Tubercular Constitution: Feebleness is the marked characteristic. The person lacks vitality, is 'run-down', nervous and always tired. The face is pale and sunken, but sometimes there is the tell-tale circumscribed red patch in each cheek. The neck is long and thin. There is a history of poor circulation, the hands and feet always being cold, yet occasionally one is told of hot flushes to the head and chest.

The appetite is precocious and often breakfast cannot be eaten. There may be a strong craving for salt.

Mentally the person is of a sullen and irritable disposition, finding fault with everyone and everything around him. There is a constant desire for change and he is always wanting to go somewhere or do something different. Sometimes there is a great depression followed by a complete reversal to hope.

In some cases the mental condition is so unstable that it borders on insanity. Kent states that 'Phthisis and insanity are convertible conditions, the one falls into the other'.

Changes of weather aggravates the tubercular patient and he is very sensitive to cold and damp. Yet he feels worse in a warm room and can only breathe easily when out in the cold wind. He feels better in a storm and one can often recognise this constitution by remembering the phrase 'Storms without and storms within'.

There is usually an evening aggravation with a rise in temperature and rapid pulse. Night sweats are common to the constitution. Periodic headaches are another indication and one should note a history of a headache each weekend. The typical headache feels as if an iron band were squeezing.

In women menstrual difficulties usually take the form of being too early, too profuse and too long lasting.

Where this constitution is suspected look for the delicate skin, cold blue extremities, the long silken eyelashes, the thin neck and elongated construction and the sunken chest bones.

Psora and Sycosis: This combination does not present the destructive manifestation of the tubercular constitution. Owing to the infiltrating properties of sycosis we expect to find diseases of the nature of tumours and overgrowths. Pelvic and urinary troubles are evidenced and gout; rheumatic heart troubles; erysipelas and herpes zoster are skin manifestations. The great majority of arthritic cases are due to these combined miasms and great relief can be given to these cases with correct treatment provided the degree of deformity is not too severe.

Psora, Sycosis and Syphilis: This is, of course, the very worst combination and by far the more difficult to cure. Among its lesser results can be seen hay fever, psoriasis and lupus, but it also leads to degenerative troubles of all sorts, particularly of the vital organs such as heart, liver, kidneys and arteries.

Where this combination exists there is a strong tendency for complaints to assume a malignant form. The great increase in cancerous affections during recent years can be traced to the spread of sycosis and syphilis on the psoric backgroud. The sycotic miasm added to the tubercular constitution at once develops the malignant types of tubercular disease.

Cases exhibiting this combination of miasms present the weakness of the psoric, the destruction of the syphilitic, and the stubbornness of the sycotic and hence remedies must be selected with the greatest care, the prescription being based upon the true symptomatology of the active miasm at the time. A remedy must be chosen capable of antidoting all three of the miasms.

Read and study Chapter 31 of Roberts' *The Principles and Art of Cure by Homoeopathy*, and re-read Chapters 22—30.

USE OF THE NOSODES

There are a large number of medicines referred to in the Materia Medica which are known as 'Nosodes'. These remedies are made from morbid or disease products, from human beings and from animals. This may at first be a repellent thought but if the student will think carefully over the lessons he has learnt regarding the preparation of the Homoeopathic remedies, he will realise that by the process of potentisation or dynamisation the disease product itself is destroyed and the energy, or activity that brought it into manifestation is retained. Hahnemann himself prepared the first Nosode from matter contained in the scabies vesicle. This he called Psorinum. Since that time many others have been prepared including Syphilinum (Syphilis), Medorrhinum (Gonorrhoea), Variolinum (Smallpox), Diphtherinum (Diphtheria), Morbillium (Measles), Pertussin (Whooping Cough), and several forms of Tuberculinum. A number of others will be found on reference to your Materia Medica.

Undoubtedly there is a close connection between diseases and their micro-organisms and the allopathic profession has pursued this discovery very fully, producing many vaccines and serums which are injected directly into the blood stream of their patients. The Homoeopath, on the other hand, uses the products of disease strictly according to the Homoeopathic laws in potency by way of mouth and as indicated by the symptoms present in the patient.

The use of the Nosodes is one of the most difficult sections of Homoeopathic medication, for the aggravation created by them, even when correctly indicated can be very severe. There are very few books written on this great subject. (Dr. Allen's MATERIA MEDICA OF THE NOSODES is probably one of the best works but difficult to obtain.) We Suggest, therefore, that students would be well advised to read widely and study the Homoeopathic principles and laws before attempting any use of the nosodes. The careless use of remedies or prescribing with insufficient knowledge can only bring the whole art and science of Homoeopathy into disrepute.

The main use of the Nosodes is when there is a personal or family history of a particular disease, or certain symptoms appear in the case-taking which *suggest* a history of a particular disease.

In almost every patient suffering from a chronic ailment there is either a history of some actual disease which can be antidoted by the appropriate nosode, or some latent disease. Where latent disease is suspected, and study of the lessons on the Chronic Miasms should have given us the indications, then the correct nosode will often unlock the door to recovery and cure.

Let us give an example of the use of a nosode from the work of Dr. H.C. Allen, a famous pioneer Homoeopath. He quotes the case of a man of 60 who suffered obstinate acute articular rheumatism. 'He suffered excruciating agony from neuralgia. After a desperate battle for life in the first week of September he was relieved, and rose from his bed a wreck. It was expected that time and out-door life and the best hygienic measures would help him. But weeks and months passed without a change; he walked the streets leaning on a cane, bent over, muffled in wraps to his ears and looking like an old man about to fall into the grave. Three months after my attendance I saw him pass

72 COMBINED MIASMS   Lesson 7

my office and considering his previous good health and robust frame the question arose 'Why does he remain in this condition?' Is there any uncured miasm, hereditary or acquired? For reasons unnecessary to mention I could not ask him.

'Dr. Swan's suggestion now occurred to me; an obstinate case of rheumatism might be due to latent gonorrhoea and Medorrhinum high will cure it; in many cases where improvement reaches a certain stage and then stops, Medorrhinum has removed the obstruction and the case progressed to a cure; and this too in cases where gonorrhoea appeared to be a most unlikely cause teaching us, if anything, the universality of latent gonorrhoea and the curative power of dynamic virus.

'His wife consulted me on other matters and said that her husband was as well as could be expected considering his age; she believed he would not do anything more, as he regarded his feeble state due to his age. However, he came next day and I gave him three doses of Medorrhinum to be taken every morning. Within ten days he returned feeling well and looking well. I then gave him one dose to be taken after some time; this was the last prescription he has required. Within a month after the Medorrhinum he dropped his cane and muffler, walked the street with a firm step, a perfectly well man having increased in weight from 140 to 212 pounds.'

An important modern field of the use of nosodes is in prophylaxis against epidemic and other acute infectious diseases. Experiments have shown that the nosode of the disease, when administered to healthy persons in small infrequent doses, will increase their resistance to that disease. For example, Morbillinum will protect against measles, Diphtherinum will protect against diphtheria and so on. When administering the nosodes in this way it is usual to give one dose of the 30th potency each week for four weeks.

TEMPERATURE

The normal temperature in man is 98.4°, this temperature remaining almost constant in health.

In disease the normal temperature may rise as high as 110°F. or sink to 90° for a time; but the risk to life is great when it passes above 106° or below 95°.

Fall of temperature may be due to many causes. It generally acompanies great loss of blood, starvation, and the collapsed condition which sometimes results from severe attacks of fever, peritonitis, and other devitalizing acute diseases. Certain chronic diseases are generally accompanied by a subnormal temperature, diabetes, Bright's disease, and myxoedema, being the most outstanding, but these diseases are for qualified medical treatment only.

Rise in temperature is a characteristic for acute diseases. Injuries to the nervous system, even unpleasant sensations in children and nervous people, may have a similar effect. A rapid rise in temperature in a person gravely ill is to be considered a most ominous sign. A high temperature in some acute diseases is, however, a much less serious feature than in others. For example, in pneumonia, a temperature of 105° is not infrequent, whilst in rheumatic fever and diphtheria the temperature generally ranges between 101° and 103°. But should the temperature go higher than the expected maximum in these cases, it is to be regarded as a very grave sign.

In most diseases the temperature gradually abates as the patient recovers, but in others the temperature drops rapidly following a 'crisis'. For example, in pneumonia the temperature suddenly falls, perspiration breaks out, the pulse becomes slower, and the breathing quieter. Often this 'crisis' is preceded by an aggravation of all the symptoms, including a sharp rise in temperature.

The temperature is measured by a clinical thermometer which registers from 95° to 110°. Care should be taken that thermometers are sterilised after use with each patient, the mercury being well shaken down to below 96°.

If for any reason it is not possible to take the temperature in the mouth, an alternative method is to place the thermometer as high as possible in the armpit, the arm being tightly folded across the chest. In this position the thermometer should be left for at least 5 minutes in order to obtain an accurate reading.

In the case of very young children, or extremely restless patients where it is advisable and even necessary to take the temperature, the thermometer may be inserted in the rectum for five or six minutes when an accurate reading should be obtained.

RESPIRATION

The breathing of a healthy person is the normal inhaling and exhaling of air, both being equal and full. The frequency varies in individuals, but usually approximates 14—18 inspirations and 14—18 expirations a minute.

In disease conditions, especially those affecting the respiratory apparatus, we should note the degree of change from normal; whether pain is present, its position, and any sounds made by the inward or outward passage of air.

Breathlessness may be due to any condition which renders the blood impure or deficient in oxygen, and which therefore produces excessive involuntary efforts to gain more air. It is often the sign of fever or inflammatory conditions, and if associated with smallness or shortness of breath, i.e. an inadequate expansion of the lungs, it indicates a degree of obstruction. This may be due to congestion (bronchitis or inflammation of the lungs) and in a later state, to fluid in the chest cavity (pleurisy or pneumonia), or to emphysema or pressure by a tumour.

Difficult breathing is often caused by a narrowing of the air passages. This is seen especially in children in such diseases as croup, asthma, and diphtheria, when the effect is possibly very sudden and alarming.

Coughs point to various derangements according to the conditions which precede, accompany or follow them. They may be associated with direct or local inflammation of the respiratory apparatus, or with sympathetic affections of these organs, originating in other organic causes of irritation, possibly in the stomach or digestive processes generally. Coughs should then be considered with all other symptoms present in order to appreciate their significance. Any cough which tends to become chronic should lead one to a very full investigation of the case.

Pain is a very important symptom and the nature of it, (stabbing, cramping) should be noted.

In all chest conditions, rest is a most important factor. When the body is quiet, the circulation becomes slower, the pulse and respiration rates slacken, and the heart and lungs are assisted in their function.

Auscultation: This is the term applied to the method of determining the condition of certain internal organs, by the sense of hearing. Breathing sounds can be heard by placing one's ear direct on the patient's chest (direct) or by the use of a stethoscope (indirect). With direct auscultation one is enabled to judge only the condition of a relatively large area, while the stethoscope brings out greater detail at localised points.

Successful use of a stethoscope, however, calls for practical training and it is not our intention to go into the art of auscultation here. We would, however, mention briefly two common terms used to describe certain sounds when studying the respiratory function.

Rales: Sounds produced by passage of air through the bronchi which contain a secretion or are narrowed by swelling of their walls or by spasms. Either 'moist' or 'dry'. Moist rales occur in conditions such as bronchitis, pneumonia, tuberculosis, pulmonary congestion etc. They can be distinguished as a bubbling or crackling sound usually appearing at the end of the inspiration. Dry rales are heard where the bronchial tubes have been narrowed as a result of inflammation of spasm (asthma), and contain a thin tenacious secretion. The act of breathing produces squeaking or groaning sounds. Sounds produced in the larger bronchial tubes are deep-toned, those in the finer tubes, piping and squeaking and whistling. These rales are often termed 'musical' on account of the different tones, produced, and are usually loudest at the end of the expiration.

Friction Fremitus: A grating feeling communicated to the hand by the movements of lungs when the membrane covering them is roughened, as in pleurisy. This sound can also be heard as a superficial rough rubbing which occurs only with respiration and ceasing when the breath is held. The quality of the sounds vary greatly; they may be grating, rubbing, rasping, and creaking.

BAPTISIA

Characteristics

Face dark red, purple; the darker red the more Baptisia. Expression besotted. Mind is confused and therefore it feels as if body is scattered about bed and he cannot collect the pieces. All discharges very offensive. Great prostration with aching and soreness all over; in whatever position the patient lies the parts rested upon feel sore and bruised. (Compare this remedy with Arnica.)

Mind:	Stupor, falls asleep whilst being spoken to. Mentally restless but cannot move.
Head:	Dull, heavy, pressive. Frontal headache with pressure at root of nose. Soreness worse stooping.
Face:	Flushed, dusky, besotted.
Mouth:	Filthy taste. Putrid, offensive breath.
Throat:	Pain and soreness of fauces. Can only swallow water. Dark putrid ulcers. Dysphagia worse swallowing liquids.
Respiratory:	Difficult breathing worse 6 p.m. Craves fresh air. Cough worse 6 p.m.
Neck and Back:	Stiffness and tenderness in neck muscles worse moving head. Aching of parts lain on worse night from 2 a.m.
Modalities:	Worse on waking; worse walking; worse open air; worse cold wind; worse Autumn or hot weather.

This remedy is almost a specific in gastric flue and epidemic influenza.

EUPERTORIUM PERF.

Characteristics

Intense aching all over the body deep in the bones, before a chill. Chill 7—9 a.m. Vomiting of bile between chill and heat.

This is another remedy which does excellent work in influenza providing the symptoms agree.

Dr. Hale describes the typical fever thus:

'The chill is nearly always in the morning and is preceded for several hours by thirst, soreness and aching of the bones. The thirst continues during the chill and heat. The chill is attended by nausea, vomiting of bile, intense aching and soreness in the flesh of the extremities and often all over the body. These symptoms continue during the heat, especially vomiting which is often painful and incessant. The heat is apt to be prolonged until evening or into the night and may be followed or not by sweat (with chilliness).

Mind:	Despondency; very restless.
Nose:	Coryza with sneezing; aching in every bone.
Stomach:	Vomiting of bile with trembling and great nausea causing great prostration.
Respiratory:	Hoarseness worse morning. Soreness of chest.
Back:	Aching pains as from bruise.
Limbs:	Aching deep in bones with soreness of flesh. Intense soreness and aching of limbs as if bruised or beaten. Compare this with Arnica.
Modalities:	Motion aggravated; changing position even slightly brings chilliness down back.

HEPAR SULPHURIS

Characteristics

Extremely sensitive mentally and especially physically to a draught of air — to least touch — and to pain which becomes so intolerable at times as to cause fainting.

Great tendency to suppurations — even slight injuries or scratches suppurate.

Mind:	Irritable and difficult to get along with. Slightest cause irritates with hasty speech and anger. Child outrageously cross.
Throat:	Choking worse cold air. Sensation of splinter or fishbone in throat.
Stomach:	Longing for acid foods.
Respiratory:	Whistling breathing worse least cold air. Cough worse least cold air. Croup — this remedy is very often needed after Aconite but only if the child is sweaty and weak and worse least cold air. Croup with rather loose cough with wheezing and rattling. As if mucus would come up but it does not — worse early morning.
Modalities:	Worse 6—7 p.m. Sudden weakness daily. Worse cold air.

This patient often wears an overcoat in hot weather. Pains are throbbing and stabbing. Discharge from all parts of body smell like old cheese or sour.

Note that the nose is stopped up every time the patient goes into the cold air.

Hepar Sulph. stands mid-way between Calc. Carb and Sulphur and the strongest characteristic is its hypersensitiveness to touch, pain and cold air. The patient can faint from pain even though it is slight. If there are inflammations, swellings or even skin eruptions the patient cannot bear to have them touched or even have cold air blow on them.

When pus is about to form, or has already formed, Hepar will hasten the discharge and help the healing.

Hepar Sulph. helps in respiratory conditions where there is chronic catarrh and the nose gets stopped up each time the patient goes out into the cold air, and is better in warm room.

It is excellent for croup when symptoms are worse by least cold air. In chronic asthma Hepar is the remedy when worse dry cold air and better damp air. Nash says he knows of no other remedy that has amelioration so strongly in damp weather as Hepar.

Hepar helps chronic dyspepsia when there is a craving for acid things — this is often accompanied by diarrhoea which is sour. The stool too is sour.

Compare Hepar with Silica as they have many symptoms in common. Dr. Farrington says: 'Hepar promotes and regulates suppuration in a remarkable manner (second only to Silica) but is generally required at an earlier stage than Silica'. Their mentalities, however, are as wide apart as poles. Dr. Tyler says: 'Silica, with its want of self confidence, its lack of 'grit'; its timidity; its suffering from anticipation — as when having to appear in public — Hepar — sensitive beyond all bounds of reason; irritable, impetuous. Sensitive to draughts, to air, ulcers so sensitive that they cannot bear the slighest touch — sensitive mentally, even to sudden murderous impulses.'

Allen says: 'The skin eruptions of Sulphur are dry, itching and not sensitive to touch; while in Hepar the skin is unhealthy, suppurating moist and intensely sensitive to touch.

Hepar is a great remedy for ears and threatening mastoid.

Kent says: 'Sweating all night without relief belongs to a great many complaints of Hepar. Inspiring cold air will increase the cough and putting the hand out of bed will increase the pain in the larynx or cough. Putting the hand or foot out of bed is a general aggravation of all the complaints of Hepar.

'The mind takes part in this oversensitiveness, and manifests iself by a state of extreme irritability. Every little thing that disturbs the patient makes him intensely angry and abusive and impulsive. The impulses will overwhelm him and make him wish to kill his best friend in an instant. Impulses also that are without cause sometimes crop out of Hepar. Impulses to do violence . . . to burn . . . to destroy. . .'

There may be dreams of fire and the pains are worse at night.

There are often habitual bronchial catarrhs with loud rattling mucus.

There is sometimes hasty speech and hasty drinking.

The sweat is often cold, clammy and offensive.

TEST PAPER No. 7

These questions should be answered only when the student feels confident that the lesson has been mastered. There should be no reference to books as this would defeat the object.

1. What miasms make up the Tubercular constitution?
2. How would you proceed to treat a patient suffering from all three miasms?
3. What is a Nosode, and when should it be used?
4. What are the chief characteristics of Hepar Sulph?

Lesson 8

THE PHYSICIAN'S PURPOSE

'The physician has no higher aim than to make sick folk well, to pursue what is called the Art of Healing.

'The physician's first duty is to enquire into the whole condition of the patient: the cause of the disease, his mode of life, the nature of his mind, the tone and character of his sentiments, his physical constitution, and especially the symptoms of his disease . . . according to the rules in the Organon.'

Thus Hahnemann summed up the essentials necessary before the Homoeopathic method of prescribing could be applied successfully, for the treatment of disease.

Let us endeavour to follow Hahnemann's instructions by studying the patient — the sick person. Here we will concern ourselves mainly with his condition — the cause of the disease, his mode of life and habits.

The condition of the Patient:

Hahnemann uses this phrase in a comprehensive manner to include all agents which may have influenced the patient's life and led to his present state. Apart from the particular symptoms of which the patient now complains we must know something of his:

1 Past History: Details of his past life; any serious illness, injury, operation, or experience which may have a bearing on the present condition.

2. Family History: Details of the health of other members of his family, and what diseases (if any) appear to recur in the family.

3. Occupational History: Type of occupation and what special stresses are placed on the patient by his employment.

4. Habits: What is his daily routine.

5. Social History: Details of personal life and the emotional factors which influence it.

Past History:
The recording of the past history falls into three main groups:

1.   Places of residence
2.   Illness suffered, and
3.   Unpleasant experiences.

1.   The place of birth should be noted and where the patient has since lived. If he has at any time been in tropical countries special enquiry should be made relative to any tropical diseases from which he may have suffered.

2.   A record of previous illnesses, operations and injuries, is next considered. What was the recovery from these? When noted in chronological order, the practitioner can visualise the progress of a disease, or tendency to a certain disease. The number of vaccinations and inoculations should also be recorded as these may well have had a profound effect upon the constitution. Where any doubt arises as to the name of a previous illness the symptoms experienced should be noted. Under this heading, it will be noted whether the patient has led an active, robust life, or whether he has been of a weakly constitution and therefore spent much of his time in sedentary occupation and hobbies.

3.   'Unpleasant experiences' covers many possibilities. Severe shocks, disappointments, griefs, war-time services are but a few of the experiences from which a person may have suffered. Special note of any circumstance, should be made when the patient states 'I have never been well since. . .' Such a remark is often made concerning the recovery from a severe illness, or when the person has suffered acutely from the loss of a loved one and so on. Similarly, consider the many forms of neuroses following war-time bombing or shell-shock. Disease has a beginning and only by diligent enquiry can we ascertain the true cause.

Family History:
The family history is of great importance to the homoeopathic prescriber as it shows the inherited constitution of the

patient and gives a general impression of the health of the patient's forebears. Some families show a definite tendency toward emotional instability; others are characteristically placid or stolid. Heart, kidney, nervous or mental diseases show a tendency to appear in members of the same family and furthermore, syphilis or tuberculosis in a family offers the hazard of contact-infection.

Special attention should be paid to the general health, habits, or particular diseases of the parents, brothers, sisters, grand-parents, uncles and aunts, and even cousins if considered necessary.

Occupational History:

This should establish the exact nature of the patient's work— what he does, and how he does it. One should have in mind the possibility of an occupational disease, some common hazards being among the following:

1. Exposure to dust or filings: Miners, metal and stone-workers, millers, seedsmen.

2. Toxic chemicals: Plumbers, house-painters, printers and workers in china and earthenware are especially exposed to lead poisoning. Similarly garage-mechanics are constantly in the fumes of carbon-monoxide, rubber workers with benzol and so on.

3. Abnormal temperature: Furnacemen, workers in cold storage plants etc.

4. Noise: Nervous affections (neuroses) are produced as a result of constant noise. Those exposed especially to this irritant are engineers, riveters and boilermakers.

One can assess from the patient's occupation whether it is sedentary or active, and whether it is dependent on mental or physical activity. Persons employed in sedentary occupations tend to suffer from digestive complaints, stomach and liver affections. Associated with mental activity is a tendency to nervous complaints.

Habits:

Mental and physical fatigue, unwise food and eating habits and the immoderate use of tea, coffee, alcohol, or the taking of drugs are often the basis of sickness in these modern times. It is therefore, necessary to obtain a *detailed* picture of the patient's daily routine as it is unlikely that he will admit that he is overworked or indulges to excess in any one thing.

The prescriber must form his own opinion on the basis of the actual facts and not on the patient's interpretation of them. Close questioning should be made as to the time of rising; how much time is allowed for eating breakfast; whether a natural urge to evacuate the bowel is suppressed until a more convenient time; what is the routine at the place of employment; what kind of lunch does he have; does he keep late hours; how he sleeps, whether he has to rely on sleeping pills.

We must also enquire as to food and drink. What constitutes for him a typical breakfast, lunch and dinner; does he eat or drink between meals; how many cigarettes are smoked each day; what drugs are taken and why; how much alcohol is taken; (here it may be necessary to refer to a member of the family or close friend if it is suspected that the patient is addicted to drinking).

Lastly, the patient's hobbies. Does he play any strenuous games; what form does his relaxation take?

Social History:

The evaluation of mental symptoms have always played a big part in homoeopathic practice and it has been proved that emotional disturbances often produce symptoms suggestive of serious organic disease. The mental state influences health by affecting the course of organic disease. For example, worry is often the predisposing cause of chronic indigestion and gastric ulcers.

In order to obtain a clear picture of the patient's emotional status it is necessary to know something of his character and his adjustment to life. One should know of his family, business, financial and sex problems. To obtain such knowledge requires great skill on the part of the prescriber and will prove extremely difficult unless the patient has absolute confidence in him and looks upon him as a friend who can be trusted.

The prescriber must, therefore, be without prejudice and view everything mentioned from the patient's standpoint. He must never express surprise or disapproval as that would create a barrier immediately. His questions must be framed in such a way that the patient does not feel the practitioner is merely inquisitive.

Questions similar to the following give us the social background to the case. Is he happy or depressed; is he satisfied with his lot in life; does he lack friends; has he any fears; does he like his work; what financial worries has he; is his salary sufficient to support him and his family; is his married life happy and normal.

Sex problems are the most difficult of all. An unhappy married life, or intense bitterness in the unmarried, can be the source of untold misery and consequent illness. A sympathetic aproach to this delicate subject will create a response, if not at the first interview, at some later date.

On the ability to understand the patient rests the ability to treat the case.

TAKING THE CASE

This is undoubtedly one of the most difficult parts of Homoeopathic treatment but it is essential that the art of case-taking be understood. Unless the case is taken properly it is impossible to find the remedy and help the patient.

REMEMBER THE PRACTITIONER NEEDS TO GET A PICTURE OF THE PATIENT THAT IS DIFFERENT FROM HIS NORM, CAUSED BY HIS SICKNESS.

The Written Record:

It is absolutely essential to have a written record of every case for symptom analysis and reference later, in order to judge whether improvement is taking place.

To be sure that no details are missed it is helpful to use a case-sheet upon which various headings have been written. When the patient has told all he can of his illness it is then up to the practitioner to fill out the picture by following up the patient's statements, making sure that no important matter has been overlooked.

Meeting the Patient:

At the initial interview we must gain the patient's confidence. If the interview is taking place in your own home it is assumed that you will show him into a quiet room where you will not be disturbed. You will, of course, see that he is comfortably seated. He should face the light in order that he may be closely observed. Remember some people will be extremely sensitive about relating intimate details of themselves and it is important to know whether they are being evasive or truthful. But be careful to distinguish the difference between embarrassment and deliberate evasion.

The attitude of the practitioner should be one of close attention. He should observe how the patient sits — whether he is restless, despondent; the colour of his eyes, hair and face. A general impression of his constitution and temperament may be formed. When he shook hands, was his hand dry or moist, hot or cold?

The Patient Talks:

Let the patient relate *in his own words* the details of his sickness. He should not be interrupted unless there is some point which is not clear. This procedure should be continued until it is quite apparent that no more can be gained without closer questioning.

The practitioner must go through the whole written record and if points are not clear encourage the patient to qualify his statements. For example, he complains of a cough; he must be asked how long he has had it, when it is worse, when better, if there is any pain, where does he feel the pain, what is the character of the pain, and in this way the symptom picture is built up.

The following will further illustrate this point:

Time: At what time of the day or night is the patient worse.

Place: What is the exact position of any pain or discomfort.

Pain or Discomfort: (these questions should be repeated respecting every pain or discomfort mentioned).

1.   You refer to a pain in your. . . At what time of the day or night would you say this pain is worse.

2.   When do you get relief from the pain.

3.   In what sort of weather is the pain worse (cold, hot, dry, wet).

4. What do you notice about the pain when the weather changes from, say, dry to wet — or vice versa.

5. How does warmth affect the pain (bed, fire, room etc.).

6. How does movement (of the arm, leg etc.) affect the pain.

7. What effect does rubbing of the part have on the pain.

8. How does pressure affect the pain. (Pressure of a hat, or clothes generally. Better loosening clothing).

9. Does the pain ever move to another part of your body? If so explain what happens.

General

10. How do you feel before, during and after meals.

11. Have you a good appetite, how do you feel if you go without a meal.

12. Are you a thirsty person — do you prefer hot or cold drinks.

13. At what time of the day or night do you feel worse.

14. What sort of weather do you dislike most — (cold, hot, dry, wet).

15. How do you feel when the weather changes. (Cold to hot etc.)

16. How do you feel before, during and after a storm.

17. Do you like warmth in general, warmth of the bed, of the room, of the fire.

18. Are you affected by draughts of air and changes in temperature.

19. In what position do you get most relief — sitting, standing, lying.

20. What vaccinations have you had; were there any noticeable reactions from them.

21. How do you feel at the seaside.

22. Do you take colds in winter or in other seasons.

23. How do collars, belts and tight clothing affect you.

24. What relief do you get by moving about, by walking.

25. How do you feel when riding in a vehicle.

26. Some people perspire a great deal. Would you say that you perspire more than a normal amount. Where particularly. Any odour.

Food Cravings and Aversions: (See under: Stomach — Appetite perverted etc.)

27. What is the kind of food for which you have a marked craving or aversion, or what are those that make you sick or you cannot eat. (Sweets, pastry, rich food etc.)

28. How much salt do you need for your taste. Pepper, mustard, pickles, sauces etc.

29. How much sugar do you like in your tea, puddings, etc.

30. How many sweets do you eat in a day.

Sleep: (See under Nervous System, Insomnia, Position Restlessness, Dreams etc.)

31. In which position do you sleep.

32. How many pillows do you have.

33. Have you ever been told that you talk, laugh, shriek etc., in your sleep.

34. At what time do you wake up. What disturbs your sleep.

35. Do you dream; do you have recurring dreams.

Mental: (See: Emotions, Fears etc.)

36. Have you at any time in your life experienced any mental shocks, bad news, good news, disappointments.

37. Do you like sympathy.

38. Do you like entertaining friends, or being entertained, or do you prefer to be alone.

39. Do you weep easily and, if so, on what occasions?

40. At what time in the 24 hours do you feel depressed, sad, or pessimistic.

41. In what circumstances do you feel jealous.

42. When and on what occasins do you you feel frightened or
    anxious (Darkness, being alone, death etc.)

43. Some people are very tidy, others not so tidy. Would you
    say you were a very tidy person or otherwise.

Menses: (See under Female Sexual System — Menstruation
etc.)

44. At what age did menstruation begin.

45. How frequent are the menstrual periods.

46. Do you have pain with the periods. If so describe the pain
    and what relieves it.

47. What is the duration, abundance, colour, odour. Are there
    any clots.

48. At what hour in the 24 hours is the flow greatest. Daytime
    or at night when resting.

49. Do you have any discharge at any other time. Describe its
    character (colour, consistency, odour etc.)

The following questions may also be helpful but each case
must be dealt with individually:

Type of pain: Whether it is a dull ache, stinging, burning, stab-
    bing, shooting.
Weather: In what sort of weather is he better or worse. Do
    changes in the weather affect him.
Thermic Reaction: How does he react to heat and cold. Simi-
    larly are his pains better in heat or cold. Reaction to the heat
    of the fire, draughts of air, etc., also come under this heading.
Possible Causation: What does the patient think caused his
    present indisposition.
Modalities: Conditions in general which aggravate or amelio-
    rate his condition, such as movement, rest, etc.
Sensations: Whether the patient has any unusual sensations,
    such as a feeling of wearing damp stockings, or that he must
    walk carefully as his legs feel brittle and may break.
Sleep and Dreams: The kind of sleep. The time of waking. Does
    he have recurrent dreams of a special nature.
Emotional Reaction: How does he react to sympathy, waiting,
    disappointments. etc.

Temperament: This is closely linked with the emotional
reaction. This part should always be left until last when the
complete confidence of the patient has been gained. The
questioning must be made very tactfully. One must judge
whether the patient is likely to be of a placid or irritable
disposition, full of life or morose, jealous in nature, sensitive
etc.

Some Mistakes:
When questioning the patient it is essential *not* to ask:

1. Leading questions which suggest answers, such as 'Does a
    cold bandage improve your headache'. This would be
    better — 'In what circumstances do you get relief from
    your headache?'

2. Direct questions. These will nearly always be answered by
    'yes' or 'no' and such an answer is quite valueless and
    should not be included in the record.

3. When a patient tells a few of his symptoms, a remedy
    sometimes comes to mind and it is very difficult not to ask
    questions which will lead the patient to give symptoms
    that may agree with the remedy already thought of. This
    type of question must be avoided.

4. Alternating questions, or skipping from symptom to
    symptom. When a patient is telling you of the pains, in
    say, his arms, keep to that subject and thoroughly exhaust
    every modality and detail possible before passing on to
    something else. Skipping from symptom to symptom con-
    fuses the patient and important questions may be for-
    gotten.

DO NOT be biased when taking the case. For instance, if the
case is similar to a previous one, it will be a temptation to
consider the same remedy. This will lead to fitting the case to
the remedy which may not be correct. Have no remedy in mind
until the details have been ascertained.

Hahnemann suggested the following method should be
adopted:

'The patient details his sufferings. The persons who are
about him relate what he has complained of, how he has be-
haved himself, and all that they have remarked in him.

The Physician sees, hears and observes with his other senses whatever there is *changed and extraordinary* in the patient. He writes all this down in the very words which the latter and the persons around him make use of.

'He permits them to continue speaking to the end without interruption, except where they wander into useless digressions, taking care to exhort them at the commencement to speak slowly that he may be enabled to follow them in taking down whatever he deems necessary.'

Hahnemann then suggests three approaches:

1. Listening to the patient.

2. Listening to those around the patient and

3. Observation.

We have dealt in some detail with the first instruction, and reference has been made to the patient's appearance. Let us consider this last instruction a little further. The patient is a middle-aged lady. She comes slowly into the room and although it is a warm day, she is wearing a coat. She sinks into th chair and lines of anxiety are apparent across her forehead. A small piece of cotton has settled on her coat; very carefully she picks it off and looks round for a receptacle in which to place it. All this may seem commonplace, but nevertheless it is possible that these observations will suggest Arsenicum. This may be noted on the record sheet for reference later — but the observation must not bias the practitioner towards that remedy.

Hahnemann's other instruction was to question those about the patient. If after much questioning the necessary facts are still not obtained, then, if possible, it is often useful to question the wife, or husband, or anyone who can give a better insight into the patient's condition. Temper their comments with commonsense however, as an anxious wife, for example, may exaggerate certain symptoms in her desire to be helpful.

Read and Study Chapter 8 of Roberts' *The Principles and Art of Cure by Homoeopathy*

BRYONIA

Characteristics:
Worse by all movements. Better pressure (or better by lying

on painful side.) Dryness of mucous membranes.

Mind: Great irritability with bouts of bad temper. Anxiety better in open air.

Head: Vertigo, faintness and nausea from raising head from pillow. Pains full, frontal, splitting or bursting, worse movement, stooping, coughing, opening or moving the eyes, in hot weather; better hard pressure.

Mouth: Dry with great thirst, for large quantities. Sour or bitter taste better after eating. Lips dry, parched, cracked.

Throat: Dry.

Stomach: Sour. Food lies in epigastrium like a stone, better bringing up wind; better eructations of tasteless gas. Pain worse breathing deeply, worse. coughing. Pains better passing flatus. Colic better walking. Nausea worse rising up from bed.

Stools: Hard and dry. Patient is often constipated. Stools large as if burnt; crumbling.

Chest: Stitching pain on coughing; patient wants to hold his chest as pressure gives relief. Breathing deeply aggravates Cough hard, dry, racking, worse coming from open air into a warm room.

Limbs: Stitching and tearing pains often in joint, better pressure or lying on painful side. Pale swellings, worse slight touch or least motion.

Fever: Chilliness worse warm room; better open air; better warm drinks; worse 9 p.m.

Modalities: Worse all movement; warmth and warm rooms; evening 9 p.m. Better rest; hard pressure; drinking large quantities.

Complaints from taking cold or getting hot in summer; from cold drinks in hot weather. Complaints when warm weather sets in after cold days. Complaints from cold winds.

One of the chief characteristics of this remedy is *Aggravation from any motion,* and a corresponding relief from absolute rest, either mental or physical. Other modalities are: Worse in warm weather after cold; and better from quiet and lying on painful side (in other words — *Better for pressure*).

Dryness runs all through the remedy; dry lips, a dry mouth; the patient will want drinks in large quantities, at long intervals. He will probably be constipated, with hard dry stools (as if burnt). His cough will be dry, hard, racking, with scanty expectoration.

Nash stated Bryonia to be 'Suitable to dry nervous slender persons of irritable disposition and rheumatic tendency'.

He also said 'It makes no difference what the name of the disease, if the patient feels greatly improved by lying still, and suffers greatly on slightest motion; and the more and longer he moves the more he suffers, Bryonia is the first remedy to be thought of, and there must be very strong contra-indications along other lines that will rule it out. Nor does it make any difference what organ or tissue is the seat of the disease, mucous, serous or muscular, the same rule applies.'

For all gastric conditions study Bryonia, Nux Vomica and Pulsatilla together and if Bryonia is the remedy there will be some of the outstanding symptoms mentioned above.

With constipation, there is no desire to go to stool; or there may be diarrhoea worse in the mornings on beginning to move. Urine is dark and scanty.

The pains of Bryonia are stitching and sticking, worse by movement and at night. The pains can be deep in the brain, in head, eyes, ears — in fact all pains of the Bryonia patient have this stitching and sticking characteristic, and they are all worse on motion and better for pressure.

Bryonia is a great East wind remedy. Patients needing this remedy have acute sufferings after exposure to cold, dry, East winds.

Mentally, Bryonia has great anxiety — anxiety about the future — and about the everyday concerns of life. Very ill-humoured, morose, everything puts him out of humour.

Dr. Tyler says 'And now, to sum up — If you get a patient with severe stitching pains, worse for the slightest movement; worse for sitting up; better for pressure; very thirsty for long drinks of cold water; very irritable; angry and not only angry but with sufferings increased by being disturbed mentally or physically; white tongue; in delirium 'wants to go home' (even if they are at home); busy in his dreams and in delirium with his everyday business, you can administer Bryonia and — bet on the result!'

RHUS TOXICODENDRON

Characteristics

Great restlessness — changes position often and this gives temporary relief. Lameness and stiffness on beginning to move after rest; on getting up in the morning; better continued motion. Triangular red tip of tongue.

Mind: Extreme restlessness, with continued change of position. Great apprehension at night, cannot remain in bed.

Face: Jaws crack when chewing. Tongue coated, except red triangular space at tip.

Back: Pain and stiffness in small of back, better motion, or lying on something hard.

Extremities: This remedy acts on fibrous tissue. Swelling and stiffness of joints from sprains, overlifting or over stretching. This may also involve ligaments, tendons and membranes of joints. Rheumatic pains in limbs, also with numbness and tingling, joints weak or stiff, worse on beginning to move and in damp weather, better from continued motion.

Skin: Itching intense. Urticaria. Burning eczematous eruptions with tendency to scale formation. Care should be used when prescribing Rhus Tox for any skin eruption as it can cause an aggravation.

Modalities: Worse (lameness, stiffness and pain) on first moving or after rest, on rising from bed in the morning. Better continued motion. The condition needing this remedy may be caused by strains, over lifting, severe muscular exercise, exposure to cold, especially wet cold.

URTICA URENS

This remedy is included for the treatment of burns and scalds, and it should be in every kitchen.

For slight burns, such as when a housewife catches her arm or hand on the hot stove, apply Urtica Urens mother tincture once or twice and the burning and stinging will go in a very short time.

For a more serious burn, a pad should be rung out in a solution of 6 drops of Urtica Urens mother tincture to a quarter of a pint of water (warm or cold). Cover the burn with this to keep out the air and bandage. At intervals when the pad dries, pour on more tincture without removing the pad from the wound.

Give Urtica Urens 30 at the same time — 2 pills every hour for three doses and then a dose when needed, i.e. when the pain returns.

TEST PAPER No. 8

These questions should be answered only when the student feels confident that the lesson has been mastered. There should be no reference to books as this would defeat the object.

1. What factors would you take into consideration when interviewing a patient for the first time.

2. Prepare an imaginary case paper for a nervous young man who complains of a hard and painful cough.

3. What must you avoid when interviewing a patient and why.

4. Name four modalities of Bryonia.

Lesson 9

AN ANALYSIS OF SYMPTOMS

'Since diseases, as dynamic derangements of the vital character, express themselves solely by alteration of the sensations and
functions of our organism, this alone can be the object of
treatment in every case of disease. For, on the removal of all
morbid symptoms nothing remains but health.'

'Nobody has ever seen 'Anaemia', 'Scarlatina' or a 'Headache', stalking abroad as a separate entity. *Symptoms are the
language in which* the disturbing forces, which we know as *disease,
speak to us.*'

Thus Hahnemann and Clarke describe symptoms — the
language of nature telling of the internal disturbance of the sick
person. From these quotations we realise:

1. That disease cannot be recognised except by its morbid
   signs and symptoms.

2. Disease can manifest itself in many different forms and
   under different conditions.

The problem, then, is how to find the remedy which will
extinguish a disease manifesting itself to our senses by these
morbid signs and symptoms. It is essential to consider the
following points:

1. A selection must be made from the mass of symptoms
   presented, and the remedy must be based on this
   selection.

2. The symptoms presented must be graded according to
   their respective values.

3. In order to match the remedy to the symptoms it is essential to know the remedies intimately and recognise those
   symptoms which characterise the patient.

Most reliance then, should be placed upon the symptoms
which signify the individual patient, and particular attention

must be paid to those symptoms which are peculiar to or characteristic of the patient, and *not* those which are common to the disease.

For this purpose symptoms can be graded into three main groups:

1. Generals — those general to the patient as a whole.

2. Particulars — those particular, not to the patient as a whole but to some part of him.

3. Common — those which are common to all cases of a certain disease.

Generals:

These are the symptoms which are general to the patient *as a whole*. When a man is unwell, he usually refers to himself as 'I' feel this or that. For example, he states 'I cannot stand the hot weather', or 'I always feel worse in the morning'.

There are three grades of Generals:

1. *The mental symptoms,* if well-marked, are of the greatest importance, taking preference over all other indications.

This is of such importance that the mental disposition of the patient often determine the selection of the remedy which will be homoeopathic to the whole case. For example: the emotional tension and fear of death of Aconite; the feeling of brittleness of Thuja.

2. Next in importance come the *Modalities* — the reaction of the patient to bodily environment, to heat and cold, damp and dry, position, time, etc. Examples of these indications are found in the pains of Bryonia and Rhus Tox. — the one being aggravated while the other is improved by motion. Aconite is aggravated by cold East winds — Belladonna is aggravated by noise and lying down but better in a sitting position.

The times of day at which symptoms occur or are aggravated have been listed separately as these are often of great value in determining the homoeopathic remedy.

We must also bear in mind that drugs often have a more pronounced action on one side of the body than the other, and where this phenomena is observed the remedy chosen should have that same modality.

3. The third grade of Generals relate to *Desires and Aversions*. These must be recent changes and must be distinct longings and loathings. For example, when a person states that he has never drunk beer, but since he felt unwell he longs for a glass, then it is a reliable indication. But a mere like or dislike is of little value.

Particulars:

These are the symptoms which bring the person for treatment, but are of less value when finding the remedy. They are applicable only to some part of the patient, hence his remarks will be prefixed with 'My'. For example, 'My shoulder is very stiff', or 'My headache is always worse when I go out in the wind'.

It is important to remember that sometimes the generals are made up of particulars. For example, if after examining the particulars of every region it is found that there are certain symptoms running through the particulars, those symptoms become generals. For instance, the patient has a dry cough, his stool is hard and dry, he has a large thirst — when we can see that the *characteristic* symptom 'Dryness' runs through the whole case.

Common Symptoms:

These are the symptoms you would expect to find in a person with a particular complaint. For example, if the patient had a fever you would expect him to be thirsty. If the case were Scarlet Fever you would expect the rash to appear. These are diagnostic symptoms and are *useful only if qualified* in some way. For instance, the fact that a patient is thirsty as a result of his illness is of no particular value in deciding the remedy, but if it is observed that although thirsty he only takes small sips of water at any one time, then the symptom becomes qualified.

Characteristic Symptoms:

Hahnemann, in the Organon, stressed the importance of securing resemblance above all things in those symptoms which are peculiar to each individual drug. He wrote 'In search for a

Homoeopathic specific remedy . . . the more striking, singular, uncommon and peculiar (characteristic) signs and symptoms of the case of disease are chiefly and almost solely to be kept in view; for it is more particularly with these that very similar ones in the list of symptoms of the selected medicine must correspond, in order to constitute it the most suitable for effecting the cure . . . If the antitype constructed from the list of symptoms of the most suitable medicine contain those peculiar, uncommon, singular and distinguishing (characteristic) symptoms, which are to be met with in the disease to be cured in the greatest number and in the greatest similarity, this medicine is the most appropriate Homoeopathic specific remedy for this morbid state.'

Characteristic symptoms, then, are *individual* symptoms, and when studying Materia Medica one should endeavour to memorise the peculiarities of each drug which are not met with in any other and which serve consequently to individualise and give character to the drug which produces them.

Dr. Kent summed up this class of symptom graphically when he wrote: 'The things that characterise are things to make you hesitate, to make you meditate. Suppose that you have been acquainted with a large number of cases of measles, for instance, but along comes one of which you say to yourself 'That is strange, I never saw such a thing as that before in a case of measles. It is peculiar.' You hesitate, you meditate, and at once recognise it as something individual, because it is strange and rare and peculiar. You say, 'I do not know what remedy has that symptom.' Then you commence to search your repertory, or, consult those of more experience, and you find in the repertory, or upon consultation, that such a medicine has that thing as a strong feature, as a high grade symptom, and it is as peculiar in the remedy as in your patient, though you have never seen it before. You may have seen a hundred cases of measles without seeing that very thing. That peculiar thing that you see in measles relates to the patient and not to the disease, and as the sole duty of the physician is to heal the sick that peculiar thing will open the whole case to the remedy. When you find that the remedy has that symptom, along with the other symptoms, you must attach some importance to it, and when there are two or three of these peculiar symptoms they form the characteristic features.'

So we see that all symptoms have value, the more characteristic of the patient they are, the more valuable on which to prescribe.

Sometimes it is difficult to decide which are the general and which are the particular symptoms. Let us refer again to Dr. Kent:

'To distinguish between what is predicted of the patient and what is predicted of a part is an essential in the study of Materia Medica. Everything that is predicted of *the patient* is general, everthing that is predicted of *a part* is a particular. The two may be opposite and hence the student of the Materia Medica will sometimes be worried because he will find aggravation from motion and relief from motion recorded under the same remedy. It is only from the sources of the Materia Medica — i.e. the provings, and from the administration of the remedy that we may observe what is true of a part and what is true of the whole. We find at times a patient wants to be in a hot room with the head out of the window for relief of the head. In that case the head is relieved from cold and the body is relieved from heat. This is a typical symptom of Phosphorus, which has relief from cold as to the head and stomach symptoms but aggravation from cold as to its chest and body symptoms. 'I want to go out in the open air and I want to take cold things into my stomach'; but if he has chest symptoms and pain in the extremities he says: 'I want to go into the house and keep warm.' And just as we see this in patients it is so in the study of a remedy; we must discriminate.'

Finally, though of great importance, come those symptoms designated by Hahnemann as being 'Strange, rare and peculiar'. These are the symptoms which characterise *this* illness in *this* patient, whether they be generals or particulars.

Note: The student will find the word 'Keynote' mentioned in many Homoeopathic books. The word appears to have been used by Dr. H.N. Guernsey originally and refers to the characteristic symptom or symptoms of a drug. He stated: 'The keynote is only meant to state some strong characteristic symptoms and on referring to the Symptom Codex (Materia Medica), all the others will surely be there if this one is. There must be a head to everything; so in symptomatology — if the most interior or peculiar, or keynote is discernible, it will be found that all the other symptoms of the case will be also found under that remedy which gives existence to this peculiar one, if that remedy is well proven. It will be necessary, in order to prescribe efficiently, to discover in every case that which characterises one remedy above another, in every combination of symptoms that exists. There is certainly something, in every case of illness, which pre-eminently characterises that case, or causes it to differ from every other. So in the remedy to be selected, there is or must be a combination of symptoms, a peculiar combination, characteristic or, more strikingly, keynote. Strike that and all others are easily touched, attuned or sounded. There is only one keynote to any piece of music, however complicated, and that note governs all the others in the various parts, no matter how many variations, trills, accompaniments, etc.'

ANALYSIS OF THE CASE

If the case has been taken correctly the next step is to study the symptoms so that the true remedy suitable to the patient may be ascertained.

We see from the mass of detail acquired at the case-taking that the symptoms listed fall into two main groups:

1. Diagnostic: Symptoms from which the disease can be diagnosed. These are usually common symptoms which are of little value in helping to find the remedy, but the remedy finally selected must include in its pathogenesis one or more of these diagnostic symptoms in order to cover the condition completely.

2. Selective: Those symptoms which are true and characteristic symptoms of the patient and from which the curative remedy is selected. They will be found among the Mental Symptoms, Modalities, Desires and Aversions and Unusual Symptoms.

Mental Symptoms:

These are the symptoms which point strongly to the mentality of the individual and can be divided into three grades:
1. The Will.

2. Perversions of Understanding and
3. Perversions of Memory.

1. In sickness the patient's nature often becomes changed
and the mental symptoms show up strongly. For example,
the patient may become very irritable, quarrelsome and
spiteful; he may turn from those nearest and dearest to
him; become tearful; or dislike sympathy. These
symptoms may be very difficult to obtain when taking the
case as the patient may try to hide them as much as
possible. (A man will hardly confess to being extremely
irritable; yet his wife may take the practitioner aside and
whisper to him 'Please, can you do something about his
temper!) Other first-grade mentals include such
symptoms as result from grief, disappointed love, bad
news, jealousy.

2. Perversions of understanding are manifested in delusions,
hallucinations, dullness of comprehension, clairvoyant
states, imbecility.

3. Perversions of memory include symptoms such as absent
mindedness, mistakes in writing and speech, failure to
remember names, inability to concentrate.

*Whenever the mental symptoms are marked, especially if changed
from normal, they are of the utmost importance to an analysis of the
case. The selected remedy must include the mental symptoms to be
curative.*

Dr. Kent illustrated the above when he wrote: 'Irritability
and mental depression run through a great many remedies, and
form the centre around which revolve all the mental symptoms
in some cases. The reason that these are more interior than
some other symptoms of the mind is that these relate to the
affections themselves. The mental symptoms can be classified
in a remedy. The things that relate to the memory are not so
important as the things that relate to the intelligence, and the
things that relate to the intelligence are not so important as the
things that relate to the affections or desires or aversions.

'We see in a state of irritabiity that the patient is not irritable
while doing the things he desires to do; if he wants to be talked

to, for instance, you do not discover his irritability while talking to him. You never discover he is irritable if you do the things he wants you to do. But just as soon as you do something he does not want, this irritability, or disturbance of the will is brought on, and this is the very innermost of the man's state, that which he wishes belongs to that which he wills, and the things that relate to what he wills are the most important things in every proving. You may say that an individual is sad, but he is sad because he lacks something that he wants; he desires something which he has not and becomes sad for it; sadness may go on to such an extent that the mind is in confusion.'

Modalities:

These are influences which aggravate or ameliorate the whole person, or the particular complaint or organ. They are found in the answers to questions relative to the time of day or night, reaction to temperature, weather, motion, position, eating, menstruation in females etc. Examples are the pains of Rhus Tox., improved by continued movement, those of Bryonia aggravated. Arsenicum is worse after midnight, while Lycopodium is worse between 4 p.m. and 8 p.m.

Modalities are marked in Homoeopathic books by the sign:

     <   Worse or aggravated by

     >   Better or ameliorated by

Unusual Symptoms:

These constitute what Hahnemann termed 'Strange, Rare and Peculiar,' and comprise all those symptoms which cannot be explained. For example, if a person has a sore throat it would be reasonable for him to desire soothing fluids only. If then the person states that his throat feels better from swallowing solids, that is unusual and search must be made to find whether any remedy has that symptom in its pathogenesis.

Dr. Kent stressed the importance of Hahnemann's instructions as follows: 'When looking over a list of symptoms, first discover three, four, five or six, or as many symptoms as exist that are strange, rare and peculiar; strange, rare and peculiar must apply to the patient himself.

'When you have settled on three or four or six remedies that have these characteristic symptoms, then find which of them is most like the rest of the patient's symptoms, common and particular.

'When you have taken a case on paper, you will settle the symptoms that *cannot* be omitted in each individual. Get the strong, strange, peculiar symptoms, and then see to it that there are no generals in the case that oppose or contradict. For example, if you see the keynotes of Arsenicum, make sure that the patient is chilly, fearful, restless, weak, pale, must have the pictures on the wall straight, and Ars. will cure.'

The Curative Remedy:

The curative remedy, then, will be one in whose pathogenesis is found the true characteristic symptoms of the patient. In other words, all those symptoms of which the patient complains, plus the all-important peculiar characteristic and mental symptoms of the patient, must be considered. The remedy which includes these symptoms will be the correct homoeopathic one to cure the patient.

Read Chapter 9 of Roberts' *The Principles and Art of Cure by Homoeopathy*

CHINA

Characteristics

Extreme debility after excessive loss of fluids and consequent debility, (diarrhoea, vomiting, haemorrhage etc.) after prolonged strain and overwork. Great flatulence with sensation as if the abdomen were packed full; not ameliorated by eructations or passing flatus. Excessive sensitiveness, especially to light touch, draught of air. Hard pressure relieves. Worse every other day. Sweats on least exertion.

Mind: Great irritability worse at night.

Head: Pain congestive, throbbing, like many hammers on temples, better hard pressure.

Mouth: Bitter taste, even water tastes bitter.

Stomach: Total loss of appetite. Full feeling after the least food, but belching only ameliorates temporarily. Digestion is slow and China is one of the most flatulent remedies.

Stools: These patients are prone to diarrhoea which is

very debilitating. Stools acrid; undigested; watery; bilious; black; painless; profuse and putrid.

Modalities: Worse slight touch; least draught of air; every other day. Better hard pressure.

China is given mostly after loss of fluids when there is very great debility and other complaints — there may be profuse haemorrhages with faintness, loss of sight and ringing in the ears.

The modalities are: worse slight touch, least draught of air, every other day — better by hard pressure on the painful part.

When a patient is very debilitated, think of China and on taking the case you will very often find 'loss of vital fluids' such as profuse leucorrhoea.

China is a very flatulent remedy and should be compared with Carbo veg., and Lycopodium. Guernsey states 'Uncomfortable distention of the abdomen with a wish to belch up, or a sensation as if the abdomen were packed full, not in the least relieved by eructation'. The impaired digestion is shown by a tendency to diarrhoea especially from eating fruit.

Note the watery stools which are painless.

This is the drug which Hahnemann first proved to discover on what principle it so acted and the following is part of his pictue of China:

'A very small dose of China acts for hardly a couple of days but a large dose, such as employed in ordinary practice, acts for several weeks, if not got rid of by vomiting or diarrhoea and thus ejected. If the homoeopathic law be right — as it incontestably is right without any exception, and is derived from pure observation of nature, viz: that medicines can only easily, rapidly and permanently cure, where the disease-symptoms match the drug disease-symptoms discovered by the administration of the drug to healthy persons, then we find, on a consideration of the symptoms of China, that this medicine is adapted for but few diseases, but that where it is accurately indicated, owing to the immense power of its action, one single, very small dose will often effect a marvellous cure.'

He goes on to say 'I say Cure, and by this I mean a recovery undisturbed by after sufferings. Have practitioners of the ordinary stamp another, and to me unknown idea of what constitutes cure? Will they call cures the suppression by this drug of agues for which bark is unsuited? I know that almost all periodic diseases, and almost all agues, even such as are not suited to China must be suppressed and lose their periodic character by this powerful drug administered usually in enormous and oft-repeated doses; but are the poor sufferers thereby really cured? Has not their previous disease undergone a transformation into another and worse disease? Thus, they no longer complain of their paroxysms appearing on certain days and at certain hours but note the earthy complexion of their puffy faces, the dullness of their eyes! See how oppressed is their breathing, how hard and distended is their epigastrium, how tensely swollen their loins, how miserable their appetite, how perverted their taste, how oppressed and painful their stomachs by all food, how undigested and abnormal their faecal evacuations, how anxious dreamful and unrefreshing their sleep. Look how weary, how joyless, how dejected, how irritably sensitive or stupid they are, as they drag themselves about.'

And this is what China in small doses can — and does cure.

China has proved of great value to patients who after an attack of influenza crawl about feeling that they would never be well again.

CARBO VEG.

Characteristics:

Desire for air — wants to be fanned. Burning internally — cold externally. Skin cold; cold sweat. State of collapse. (Sometimes from surgical shock.) Flatulence.

Mind:	Timid; slowness; sluggish; lazy.
Head:	Vertigo after slightest movement. Pain pressive; worse warmth of bed. Pain from being overheated. Pain burning and throbbing worse breathing deeply. Pains better eructations.
Nose:	Nose feels cold.
Face:	Face flushes after drinking wine.
Stomach:	Weak digestion with enormous production of flatulence, better eructations. Excessive accumulations of gas, feels full and tense. Flatulence

worse milk. Flatulent colic worse lying. Symptoms worse wine; worse warmth, worse evening.

Respiratory: Dry, hacking cough, distressing patient. Cough worse on entering cold air from warm room. Rawness and soreness of larynx; hoarseness; worse evening; worse warm, moist weather. Loss of voice worse morning.

Limbs: Rheumatic pains better eructations. Feet and hands cold; knees cold.

Modalities: Patient is better from eructations and from being fanned. Worse morning on waking. Perspiration copious and cold.

This is a Corpse reviver and in desperate cases of collapse, where the patient is icy cold and demands to be fanned, it has saved life.

LYCOPODIUM

Characteristics:

Hunger, but a little food seems to fill stomach and causes fullness and distension of abdomen. Worse 4—8 p.m. Red sediment in urine. Right sided — or complaints go from right to left. Better warm drinks; worse cold food and drink. Fan-like movement of alae nasi (nostrils). Suddenness — sudden flashes of heat; lightning like pains; sudden satiety; pains and symptoms come and go suddenly.

Mind: Very nervous, sensitive, emotional person; apprehensive. Apprehensive of undertaking anything yet he is all right when he does it. Likes his own company but prefers somebody to be in the house in another room. Emotional and weeps when thanked.

Head: Bursting, pressing headaches. Headaches better when catarrh is worse. Worse 4—8 p.m.

Nose: Must breathe through mouth at night.

Throat: Sore right side or going from right to left. Worse 4—8 p.m. Better warm drinks. If you hear a patient complaining of a feeling as though a ball is rising into the throat from below — a dose of Lycopodium will cure.

Stomach: Patient feels very hungry but after a few mouth-
                  fuls becomes full up, bloated and uncomfortable.
                  Is distended like a drum and says 'everything I
                  eat turns to wind'. Cannot eat oysters. This is one
                  of a trio of flatulent remedies with Carbo Veg.
                  and China. China bloats the whole abdomen,
                  Carbo Veg. prefers the upper part and Lyc. the
                  lower part. China has fullness after a normal
                  meal and Lyc. after eating little.

Urinary: Sediment like red sand in urine.

Respiratory: Stitches in L chest and during inspiration. Very
                  difficult breathing.

Back: Burning between scapulae as of hot coals.

Extremities: One foot hot and the other cold.

Sleep: Patient is worse in the evening and better on
                  waking but wakens cross and irritable.

Modalities: If you have a patient with at least three of the
                  following modalities and the other symptoms of
                  the case fit then you can be sure that Lyco-
                  podium is the correct remedy.

                  Worse afternoon — Desires hot drinks

                  Worse 4 p.m.—8 p.m. — Craves sweets

                  Has Urinary troubles — Has acidity and
                  bloating and wind.

                  Better by motion, warm food and drink, in the
                  open air, being uncovered, after midnight.

Kent says 'Though classed among inert substances and
thought to be useful for rolling up allopathic pills Hahnemann
brought it into use and developed its power by attenuation. It
enters deep into the life. There is nothing about man that Lycopodium does not rouse into tumult.'

Dr. Kent explains that the Lycopodium patient wants to be
alone but likes to feel that somebody is in the next room because
he fears to be alone. He also fears death — and the dark. This
patient weeps when meeting a friend, is tired with chronic
fatigue — is forgetful, and therefore has aversion to undertaking anything new. The mind of the Lycopodium patient is
better developed than the body — they often look older than
they really are.

The Lycopodium patient anticipates things and is nearly sick until they happen; then he goes through everything feeling on top of the world. He cannot think how he can make a speech but when he gets on his feet he feels quite confident.

TEST PAPER No. 9

These questions should be answered only when the student feels confident that the lesson has been mastered. There should be no reference to books as this would defeat the object.

1. What kind of symptoms would you regard as:
   (a) General
   (b) Mental
   (c) Particular

2. Why is it wrong to prescribe only on particulars?

3. What have the three remedies Lycopodium, Carbo Veg and China in common?

4. Give four characteristics of Lycopodium.

Lesson 10

REPERTORISING

Having taken the case we must now find the remedy and our next step is to decide which one can be used as an eliminating symptom. By this we mean that where, for instance, a person states 'I cannot stand the cold weather' it is useless to consider remedies which are characterised by beng predominantly for 'hot people'. One of these remedies may seem to be well indicated but unless it presents a picture of the patient as a whole it is not the correctly indicated remedy.

Our eliminating symptom must, therefore, be:

1. An individual characteristic of the patient.

2. A selective symptom of importance — i.e. a strong modality.

3. It should have a reasonable number of remedies in the rubric so as not to limit our choice without further verification.

The eliminative symptom determines our primary list of remedies, i.e. the correct remedy will be one of those mentioned in the repertory under this particular symptom.

To illustrate these instructions let us work through the symptoms of the simple example of the acute case we have already discussed.

The character of the headache is very pronounced — splitting or bursting — and it must therefore be a strong characteristic of the chosen remedy for it to be curative. Let us use it as our eliminative symptom. Various other remedies are noted in the Repertory but for this case we shall only consider those with which you are already familiar. Bearing in mind that there is also restlessness and anxiety and a hot dry skin with a quick pulse, our choice will lie between Aconite and Belladonna. In order to decide which of these two remedies is the better indicated reference must now be made to the Materia Medica.

In the Materia Medica Pura, Hahnemann gives an example of case analysis which has been quoted many times in Homoeopathic literature. We give this example below as an illustration of how the characteristic symptoms guide unerringly to the correct remedy.

'Sch . . . a washerwoman, somewhere about forty years old, had been more than three weeks unable to earn her bread when she consulted me on September 1, 1815.

1. On any movement, especially at every step, worse on making a false step, she has a shock in the pit of the stomach, that comes as she avers, every time from the left side.

2. When she lies she feels quite well; then she has no pain anywhere, neither in the side nor at the pit of the stomach.

3. She cannot sleep after 3 a.m.

4. She relishes her food, but when she has eaten a little she feels sick.

5. Then water collects in her mouth and runs out of it like water-brash.

6. She has frequent empty eructations after every meal.

7. Her temper is passionate, disposed to anger. When the pain is severe she is covered with perspiration. The catamenia was quite regular a fortnight since.

In other respects her health is good.'

Hahnemann then describes how he decided on the indicated remedy.

'Now as regards Symptom 1, Belladonna, China and Rhus Tox., cause shooting in the pit of the stomach on making a false step, but none of them *only on movement*, as is the case here. Pulsatilla certainly causes shooting in the pit of the stomach on making a false step, but only as a rare alternating action, and has neither the same digestive derangements as occur here at 4 compared with 5 and 6, nor the same state of the disposition.

'Bryonia alone has among its chief alternating actions, as the whole list of its symptoms demonstrates, pain *from movement,* and especially shooting pains, as also stitches beneath the sternum (in the pit the stomach) on raising the arm, and on making a false step it causes shooting in other parts.

'The negative symptom 2 met with here answers especially to Bryonia; few medicines (with the exception, perhaps, of Nux Vomica and Rhus Tox., in their alternating action — neither of which, however, is suitable for the other symptoms) show a complete relief to pains during rest and when lying; Bryonia does, however, in an especial manner.

'Symptom 3 is met with in several medicines, and also in Bryonia.

'Symptom 4 is certainly, as far as regards sickness after eating, met with in several other medicines (Ignatia, Nux Vomica, Mercurius, Ferrum, Belladonna, Pulsatilla, Cantharis), but neither as constantly and commonly, nor with relish for food, as in Bryonia.

'As regards symptom 5, several medicines certainly cause a flow of water like water brash, just as well as Bryonia; the others however, do not produce symptoms similar to the remaining ones. Hence Bryonia is to be preferred to them in this particular.

'Empty eructations (of wind only) after eating (symptom 6) is found in few medicines, and in none so constantly, so commonly and to such a degree as in Bryonia.

'To 7, one of the chief symptoms in diseases (see Organon, sec. 213) is the "State of the disposition", and as Bryonia causes this symptom also in an exactly similar manner, Bryonia is for all these reasons preferred in this case to all other medicines as the homoeopathic remedy.

Thus Hahnemann decided on the one remedy which was homoeopathic to the case. He goes on to describe how the remedy was prescribed and the result:

'Now as this woman was very robust, and the force of the disease must consequently have been very considerable to prevent her, on account of the pain, doing any work, and as her vital powers, as stated, were not impaired, I gave her one of the strongest homoeopathic doses, a full drop of the undiluted juice of Bryonia root to be taken immediately, and bade her come to me again in forty-eight hours. I told my friend E. who was present, that within that time the woman would assuredly be quite cured; but he, being but half converted to homoeopathy, expressed his doubts about it. Five days afterwards he came again to learn the result, but the woman did not return then, and in fact, never came back again. I could not allay the impatience of my friend by telling him her name and that of the village where she lived, about a mile-and-a-half off, and advising him to seek her out and ascertain for himself how she was. This he did and her answer was 'What was the use of my going back? The very next day I was quite well, as I am still. I am extremely obliged to the doctor, but the likes of us have no time to leave off our work, and for three weeks previously my illness prevented me earning anything.'

The following is an example of a case taken and repertorised:

Jan. 28th 1956
Mr S. Married man, aged 56, dark, dark eyes, face yellowish and whites of eyes, called and stated:

Particulars
In the 1914/18 war went deaf in the right ear. Operated on (as it was steadily getting worse) in 1955, to remove, what the ear specialist said, was a fungus growth around the eardrum. Can only hear now with this ear with a hearing aid. The right ear which was O.K. is now so bad that he can't hear at all.

Years ago had a drawing pain in the left hip. This went and there followed in the left thigh, a sudden stab like burning pain; and after this there developed a cramping pain, which used to come on suddenly when walking. When sitting a continuous dull ache better temporarily by constantly changing position.

Now the pain commences in the left ankle, and starts with a burning pain, which moves to the left knee, and then to the thigh which is worse by heat. When the pain reaches the thigh, a sort of sudden internal explosion in the thigh takes place, which throws the leg up and is worse at night and the warmth of bed. Grinds his teeth in sleep.

He HIMSELF loathes DAMP COLD WEATHER, and is better in the warmth.

Past History
1. In the nineteen-twenties had two small hard warts, one on the left side of his forehead, the other below the larynx.

The one on the head was burnt off with nitrate of silver. The other he picked, and it eventually went.

2. As a child he fainted very easily for no reason.

3. Father was cruel and constantly used a hunting-crop on his boys.

4. Has had pleurisy worse left side.

HIMSELF

Dislikes consolation and fuss, makes him very irritable.
Impatient.
Dislikes company.
Worse room full of people.
Conscientious about trifles.
Worse greasy (fat foods).
Thirstless.
Worse external·constriction.
Occasional burning pain AFTER urination.
Fainting easily as a child.
Grinding teeth in sleep.

In searching for the remedy, as HE HIMSELF loathes Cold damp weather, we can eliminate ALL remedies which are WORSE by HEAT.

Now this is how we worked out the remedy.

Worse consolation and fuss. Ars-Bell-Calc-Phos, Hell-IGN, SEP, SIL.

Impatient. Ars, IGN, SEP, Sil.

Aversion to company. IGN, Sep.

Room full of people. Sep.

Conscientious over trifles. Sep. (low)

Worse greasy (fat) foods. Sep.

Thirstless. Sep.

Worse external constriction. Sep.

Burning after urination. Sep (low)

Fainting. SEP.

Grinding teeth in sleep. Sep. (low)

Particulars
Drawing pain in hip. Sep.

Stitching pain thigh, internally. SEP.

Burning pain. SEP.

Cramp, thigh. Sep.

Pain sudden. Sep (low)

Better motion of affected part. Sep.

Worse night. SEP.
Pain moves upwards. SEP.

Warts hard. Sep.

Warts small. Sep.

Worse left side. SEP

Face yellow. SEP

Eyes yellow. SEP.

   Sepia is therefore the most similar remedy.

PULSATILLA

Characteristics:
   Patient must have fresh air, although she is chilly. Worse in warm stuffy room. Better moving about slowly. Cannot tolerate fats or rich greasy foods. Thirstless. Changeable — pains wander; no two chills are alike; no two stools are alike; menstruation is never the same and so on.

Mind:	Patient can weep easily; affectionate but can also be very irritable.
Head:	Pains better whilst moving about slowly in cool air. Likes to sleep with head high — raised with two or three pillows.
Nose:	Discharge bland, yellow-green mucus.
Mouth:	Dry without thirst. Expectoration bitter. Burnt taste in mouth.

Better moving slowly. Worse warm stuffy rooms; worse fat and greasy foods.

Stomach: Very easily disordered by fats. Intolerance of fat and rich food.

Modalities: Better in cold air and from cold applications.

Hahnemann says 'This very powerful plant produces many symptoms in the healthy, which often corresponds to the morbid symptoms commonly met with.'

The Pulsatilla patient seeks the open air — he is always better out of doors even though he is a chilly person. The open air relieves vertigo, pains in head, eye symptoms, fluent coryza, toothache, cough etc. Walking relieves vertigo, toothache, sticking pains in stomach and liver, bruised pains in back and knees.

But the Pulsatilla patient must not get wet — this can mean colic, attacks of mucous diarrhoea, rheumatism, suppressed menses, etc. Note — the Pulsatilla patient is better for cold air, cold dry air but not wet air.

The Pulsatilla patient is not hungry, not thirsty and not constipated.

Keynotes   Aversion to fat and rich food.
Chilly yet worse for heat.
Craves the open air.
Craves movement, if in pain, either physical or mental.
Haemorrhages flow, stop and flow again.
Headaches better by tying up the head.
Wandering pains.

Although the patient needing Pulsatilla cannot stand heat, she is a chilly patient and must have air.

Pulsatilla leads all remedies 'worse from heat'.

If you come across a patient suffering from any aches, pains or discomforts, and he or she wants to move slowly in the cool air (or if she is in bed MUST have plenty of fresh air) is very tearful and cannot tolerate any fats, then PULSATILLA will cure — whatever you may call the ailment.

The disposition of Pulsatilla is almost opposite to that of Nux Vomica.

Silica is the chronic of Pulsatilla.

ALLIUM CEPA

Dr. Clarke says 'Allium Cepa covers more symptoms of the common cold than any other remedy, as the well-known effects of onions in producing tears would suggest.

Characteristics.

Symptoms worse in a warm room; better in open air; worse again on returning to warm room. Burning. Inflammation and increased secretion of mucous membrane. Neuralgic pains like a long thread. (In face, neck and head.)

Head:	Dull headache with coryza worse evening; better in open air but worse when returning to warm room. Pains in temples, occiput and down neck.
Eyes:	Flow of tears; excessive non-excoriating lachrymation of eyelids; worse evening. Burning.
Nose:	Profuse watery discharge, with sneezing, acrid, burning, excoriating nose and upper lip. Fluent coryza better in open air and worse in warm room. Worse evening and worse Spring.
Throat:	Sensation as of a lump in throat. Expectorations of a lumpy mucus through posterior nares. Burning. Pain in throat extending to ear.
Respiratory:	Tickling of larynx and constant inclination to hack in order to clear throat. Cough from inhaling cold air.
Modalities:	Worse warm room; worse evening; Better open air and motion. Damp cold wind and weather brings on colds.

TEST PAPER No. 10

This task should be undertaken only when the student feels confident that the lesson has been mastered. There should be no reference to books as this would defeat the object.

1. Write up an imaginary case history and then state which you think would be the eliminating symptom for repertorising the case, and why.

Lesson 11

ADMINISTRATION OF THE REMEDY

Having decided on the one remedy which will be homoeo-pathic to the case we must know when and how it should be administered in order to utilise its maximum effect.

A most important point to bear in mind is that in homoeo-pathic dosage a drug does not act directly on a disease, but stimulates the natural resistance of the body to the disease. If, therefore, after a single dose of the indicated remedy it becomes apparent that the natural powers have been awakened it is not only unnecessary but unwise to repeat the dose.

Hahnemann stated this as follows: *'Perceptible and continued progress of improvement* in an acute or chronic disease is a condition which, as long as it lasts, invariably *counter-indicates the repetition of any medicine whatever,* because the beneficial effect which the medicine continues to exert is aproaching its perfection. Under these circumstances every new dose of any medicine, even of the last one that proved beneficial, would disturb the process of recovery.'

Rule 1:   Never repeat while improvement is maintained.

'The same remedy may be given a second time when the improvement which the first dose had produced . . . ceases to continue . . . when it becomes evident that the medicine has ceased to act, the condition of the mind being the same as before, and no new or troublesome symptoms having made their appearance. All this would show that the same remedy is again indicated.'

Rule 2:   Repeat the same remedy only when improve-ment ceases and the symptoms return in their orignal form.

'When there comes an end to the improvement, which has gone steadily forward though not to complete recovery, a precise examination of the present improved aspect of the disease will show a small and *altered symptom-group,* to which a second dose of the former medicine would no longer be suitably homoeopathic. Another counter-force is required, more adapted to the remaining phenomena of the disease.'

Rule 3:   Change the remedy when improvement ceases and symptoms have altered.

Acute Disorders

It is characteristic of acute illness that its onset and progress is rapid ending either in recovery or death. The body resources are, therefore, being constantly called upon to expend vital energy. In order to give maximum assistance to the body at this time it is necessary to aid the vital force as frequently as possible.

'In acute diseases the time for the repetition of the proper remedy is regulated by the rate at which the disease runs its course; here it may often be necessary to repeat the medicine in twenty-four, sixteen, twelve, eight, four hours, and less, while the medicine, without originating new complaints, continues to produce uninterrupted improvement; but where this improvement is not sufficiently marked, considering the dangerous rapidity of the acute disease, the interval may be still further lessened.'

Repetition in acute cases, then, is regulated by the rate at which the disease runs its course, *provided the symptoms remain the same.*

Occasionally it will be found that in an acute case the seemingly indicated 'acute' remedy does not have the desired effect or, having at first produced an improvement, the improvement does not hold. Here there is evidence that there is some chronic background to the case which has not been sufficiently considered. Later notes will make this paragraph clearer and you will know the course of action to adopt.

Chronic Diseases

A chronic disease is characterised by its slow progress, showing little tendency towards recovery. It is therefore reasonable to assume that under treatment improvement will be governed by the same characteristic, and a return to health will be correspondingly slow.

Nevertheless, the rules apply regarding administration of the remedies, viz:

Rule No. 1:   Never repeat while improvement is maintained.

Rule No. 2:   Repeat the same remedy only when improvement ceases and the symptoms return to their original form.

Rule No. 3:   Change the remedy when improvement ceases and symptoms have altered.

REMEDY REACTION

'This eternal, universal law of Nature, that every disease is destroyed and cured through the similar artificial disease which the appropriate remedy has the tendency to excite, rests on the following proposition: that only one disease can exist in the body at any one time, and therefore one disease must yield to the other.' (Organon)

'Since diseases, as dynamic derangements of the vital character express themselves solely by alterations of the sensations and functions of our organism, that is, solely by an aggregate of cognizable symptoms, this alone can be the object of treatment in every case of disease. For, on the removal of all morbid symptoms nothing remains but health.' (Materia Medica Pura).

'To every disease the organism reacts in a special and individual way.' (Organon)

After the administration of the similar remedy it is to be expected that a reaction will take place — the greater the similarity the greater the reaction — and in simple acute cases improvement should be almost immediate. Failure to obtain quick relief shows that the remedy selected was not a near similar and the case must be re-taken.

In more serious acute cases there should still be a measure of improvement. This may not be evidenced by immediate relief of the symptoms, but may show itself by a calmer mental condition, less pain, a drop in temperature in feverish conditions, a more restful sleep and so on. Hahnemann expressed it as follows: 'The condition of the mind and the general behaviour of the patient are among the most certain signs of incipient improvement, or of aggravation, in all diseases, especially in acute ones.

Incipient improvement, however slight, is indicated by increased sense of comfort; greater tranquillity and freedom of mind; heightened courage and a return of naturalness in the feelings of the patient.

'The signs of aggravation, however slight they may be, are the opposite of the preceding, and consist in an embarrassed, helpless state of mind, while the deportment, attitude, and actions of the patient appeal to our sympathy.'

In chronic conditions relief may not come for days, or even weeks, and one must tell the patient of this fact from the outset so that he will not become discouraged. Even in these cases, however, there is often a striking improvement in the patient's mentality — he feels better in himself, though the symptoms of which he complained may be no better or even worse.

Homoeopathic Aggravation:

'Least of all, need we to be concerned when the usual customary symptoms are aggravated and show most prominently on the first days, and again on some of the following days, but gradually less and less. This so-called homoeopathic aggravation is a sign of an incipient cure (of the symptoms aggravated at present), which may be expected with certainty.' (Chronic Diseases)

Often the reaction to the remedy takes on the form of an aggravation of the symptoms present, the aggravation being usually dependent on whether the remedy was particularly well selected and the patient very sensitive to that remedy, or the potency of the remedy not quite suitable. In disease, the patient is very susceptible to a remedy which is capable of producing similar symptoms in the healthy, and as mentioned in a previous lesson, the potency should be carefully considered before administration in order to avoid, as far as possible, any severe aggravations.

Dr. Kent states: 'Whenever you find an aggravation comes quickly, is short, and has been more or less vigorous, then you will find improvement of the patient will be long . . . such is the slight aggravation of the symptoms that occurs in the first hours after the remedy in an acute sickness, or during the first few days in a chronic case.

'In acute disease we seldom see anything like striking aggravation unless the acute disease has drawn near death's door, or is very severe . . . If the disease has ultimated itself in change of tissue, then you see striking aggravations, even aggravations that cannot be recovered from.

'An aggravation of the disease means the patient is growing weaker, the symptoms are growing stronger; but the true homoeopathic aggravation, which is the aggravation of the symptoms of the patient while the patient is growing better, is something that the physician observes after a true homoeopathic prescription. The true homoeopathic aggravation I say, is when the symptoms are worse but the patient says "I feel better".' (lectures on Homoeopathic Philosophy)

From the foregoing we can now summarise as follows:

1. *No change.*
   (a)   The remedy wrongly selected or given in wrong potency.
   (b)   Slow-acting remedy.
   (c)   Patient sluggish in reacting.
2. *Steady improvement with no aggravation.*
   (a)   Remedy correct.
   (b)   No organic change and no tendency to organic disease.
3. *Short and strong aggravation followed by a slow and sure recovery.*
   (a)   Remedy correct.
   (b)   Vigorous reaction indicates that there is no structural change in the vital organs.
   (c)   A reaction to be desired as there is always a rapid improvement following a short and strong aggravation.
4. *Long and severe aggravation followed by a slow and sure recovery.*
   (a)   Remedy correct but must *not* be repeated until its action completely exhausted.
   (b)   Organic changes will have been in evidence before remedy administered. Vital force of patient low, but where the case is curable a general improvement in health will be manifest.
5. *Improvement limited.*
   (a)   Remedy correct, but where the vital organs have been much affected or after severe operations a complete

return to absolute health is not possible. Careful repetition of the remedy at infrequent intervals will keep the patient comfortable.

6. *Long aggravation followed by a slow decline of the patient.*

(a)   Usually indicates that the case is incurable. This type of reaction is only observed in advanced cases of disease where much organic destruction has already taken place.

7. *Amelioration first with aggravation after.*

(a)   An improvement appears to commence which lasts for several days, but after a week or so all the symptoms are worse than before the remedy was administered. Here the remedy selected was not sufficiently deep-acting or the case is incurable.

Allow sufficient time for the remedy to exhaust its action and retake the case. A remedy selected on the whole totality now exhibited may produce a curative reaction.

Only by careful observation of the symptom before selecting the remedy, and by careful observation of the reactions after the administration of the remedy, can one know whether satisfactory progress is being made in each individual case.

Read Chapter 14 of Roberts' *The Principles and Art of Cure by Homoeopathy*

SILICA

Characteristics:

Want of grit — moral and physical. 'What silica is to the stalk of grain in the field, it is to the human mind'.Worse anticipation. Coldness — lack of vital warmth even when taking exercise; must be wrapped up, especially head. Suppressed sweat especially of feet which is profuse and offensive. Constipation — stools protrude and then slip back again and again, weak expulsive power. Weak puny children through defective assimilation. Inflammations ending in suppuration, heals after discharge has taken place.

Mind: Want of grit, moral and physical. Nervous irritable, weak, fainthearted, yielding disposition.

Head: Vertigo ascends from nape of neck to head, worse looking up. Pain beginning in nape of neck and going up over head to eyes and settling over one eye, usually the right, better pressure and wrapping up head.

Nose: Alternate fluent and dry coryza. Acrid and corrosive mucus in nose. Coryza worse daytime.

Throat: Sore with an accumulation of mucus. Pain similar to pricking of pins. Symptoms worse evening.

Anus: Constipation, stool comes down with great difficulty; comes a little way through anus and then slips back before it can be voided.

Back: Pain in base of spine (coccyx) worse riding in car.

Limbs: Dryness in tips of fingers. Nails brittle with white spots. Feet cold. Profuse, offensive perspiration.

Skin: Sensitive — small wounds heal with difficulty and suppurate profusely.

Modalities: Worse cold, draught, motion, open air, at new moon. Better warm room, wrapping head up.

Patients needing this remedy are very sensitive to cold; they take cold very easily especially when uncovering head or feet. Better wrapping up head.

Silica is the chronic of Pulsatilla. Never use it in a high potency where there is any history of T.B.

Remember Silica expels foreign bodies so be careful if the patient has a history of any embedded shrapnel etc., which may be better undisturbed.

Dr. Tyler gives a clear picture of a Silica child as follows:

'Silica is dragged reluctantly in, not interested, not frightened. You see a pale, sickly suffering face. He doesn't get on and he doesn't thrive — is irritable and grumpy — he is always at the bottom of his class, shirks responsibility and is lacking in self assertion and self confidence. He cannot think and fix his attention on anything — he cannot read or write and yet is worried over little things he has done wrong. He gets violent attacks of headache, and complains that the back of his head is cold. Complains of bursting head and wants it warm — wants it tied up — he is always ill with the new moon — he gets bad coughs and expectorates lumpy yellow or green mucus — his nails are rough and yellow and there is a feeling of a splinter in his finger, or his finger gets red and throbs. His skin will not heal, he gets festers when he scratches himself and with every sore there is a sticking and burning pain. He is very thin. He is very cold even in a warm room and cannot sleep for cold feet — is cold up to his knees. But he sweats, especially at night. Has no appetite and is always tired. Has frightful dreams. He has a very offensive stool and the perspiration is very offensive, and his feet perspire freely — and in between the toes. His stomach is hard and swollen with lots of wind which smells.

And now, quoting from Dr. Clarke — 'A curious symptom and one of great value is this — 'Fixed ideas; the patient thinks only of pins, fears them, searches for them and counts them carefully'. This symptom helped me to make a rapid cure of post influenzal insanity in the case of a man of bad family history, one of whose sisters had become insane and drowned herself, another sister being affected with lupus. The patient's wife told me one morning that he had been looking everywhere for pins. Sil. 30 rapidly put an end to the search for pins and restored the patient to his senses. Silica has another link with insanity in its aggravation at the moon's phases; epilepsy and sleep-walking are worse at the new and full moon'.

Dr. Kent says: 'The action of Silica is slow. In the proving it takes a long time to develop the symptoms. It is suited, therefore, to complaints that develop slowly. The long acting, deep acting remedies are capable of going so thoroughly into the vital disorders that hereditary disturbances are routed out. The mental state is peculiar. The patient lacks stamina. What Silica is to the stalk of grain in the field, it is to the human mind. When the mind needs Silica it is in a state of weakness, embarrassment, dread, a state of yielding. It is the natural compliment and chronic of Pulsatilla, because of its great similarity; it is Puls. only more so, a deeper, more profound remedy.

Silica is often called the Surgeon's knife of the Homoeopath because it is the remedy used to promote suppuration.

GELSEMIUM

Characteristics:
Mentally dull and sluggish with desire to be left alone. Muscles relaxed and weak. Eyelids droop. Limbs heavy.

Thirstless. Internal and external trembling. Child suddenly starts and grasps the nurse and screams as if afraid of falling.

Mind: Mentally dull. Nervous patient. Excitement on hearing bad news. Stage fright or examination funk.

Head: Vertigo worse on sudden movement. Dull tired ache at base of brain. Wants head raised on high pillow and kept still. (Headache is often relieved by profuse flow of urine.) Also 'sick' headache, preceded by blindness — as head begins to ache blindness disappears.

Eyes: Eyelids droop.
Throat: Dryness and burning.
Chest: Sensation as if the heart would stop beating if she did not move about.

Neck and   Muscles of neck feel bruised. All muscles feel
Back: bruised.

Limbs: Trembling in all limbs; deep seated dull aching in muscles of limbs and in the joints. Trembling worse mental emotions. Trembling with fear, has to be held.

This patient complains of being so tired — he wants to lie down and rest.

Modalities: Motion aggravates most symptoms. Worse cold damp weather. Better cold open air. Worse damp weather.

          'One of the first things you hear from a patient needing Gelsemium is "Doctor I'm so tired" '.

IGNATIA

Characteristics:
This is a remedy of contraries, of symptoms which do not make sense: i.e. all throat symptoms are better swallowing someting hard like toast. Mental and physical contrariness. Changeable mood and disposition. Twitchings.

Mind: The remedy of moods; gaiety alternating with the disposition to weep. Suppressed grief with long drawn sighs, much sobbing, desires to be alone with her grief. Fears she will never sleep again. Melancholy — sits in a vacant stare. Worn out nervous patients. Hysteria. Impatient, quarrelsome, angry.

Head: Pain as if nail were driven out through the side of head, better lying on it; particularly in highly nervous and sensitive people. Headache symptoms are changeable and are worse coffee, smoking, alcohol, cold winds, change of position; better warmth, soft pressure and profuse flow of urine.

Throat: All throat symptoms are better by swallowing something hard like toast.

Stomach: Empty faint weak feeling. Weak digestion but lobster salad for supper does not upset him.

Anus: Pains sharp and stitching, shooting up into rectum, better whilst sitting.

Modalities: Better by heat and aggravated by cold.

TEST PAPER No. 11

These questions should be answered only when the student feels confident that the lesson has been mastered. There should be no reference to books as this would defeat the object.

1. When is it safe to repeat a remedy at short intervals?
2. What would you expect after giving a remedy in a chronic case if:
   (a) There was very limited improvement.
   (b) Rapid improvement after a short, sharp aggravation.
3. When is it unwise to repeat a remedy?

Describe a patient who need Silica.

Lesson 12

DRUG RELATIONSHIPS

It has been observed in proving and in clinical application that a relationship exists between certain remedies. This is because the particular drugs originate from a similar source or belong to the same botanical family or chemical group. Where this relationship exists it will be found that certain features are common to these remedies. For example, through the several Calcium drugs — the Carbonate, and Phosphate, etc., — runs th typical Calcium weakness and debility. Where Iron is the active principle in remedies, such as Aconite, Belladonna, and Ferrum Phos., there can be observed inflammatory states.

It is a good plan to study remedies in 'family' groups, noting both the points of similarity and more especially the points of difference. Dr. Nash's book *Leaders in Homoeopathic Therapeutics* will be helpful to you in this study.

Compatible Relationships

This term includes remedies which are complimentary to each other, or which follow each other well. Often certain remedies act better when prescribed in a series. For example, Pulsatilla is followed well by such remedies as Arsenicum, Lycopodium, Nux Vomica, Sepia, Silica and Sulphur.

A truly complimentary remedy is one which completes the work done by the previous remedy. For example, Sulphur completes the action of Aconite when all the good which can be expected of that remedy is exhausted. Other examples are Calc. Carb., following Belladonna; Natrum Mur., following Ignatia.

These following medicines are called the 'chronics' of the 'acutes' by some writers. Thus Ignatia is the acute and Nat. Mur., is the chronic. Ignatia is for grief but if there are deeper changes in the patient's nature and character which may only be shown after the Ignatia has been given, then Nat. Mur., is the natural compliment, providing always that all other symptom are in agreement.

Inimical Relationships

This is the opposite of the above. There is a lack of harmony between the action of the drugs when following each other in the treatment of a case. Often it is observed that inimical remedies have a similar pathogenesis and the action of the following drug spoils the action of the original prescription. An example of this can be observed where Sulphur follows Calcarea, or Rhus tox follows Apis in skin troubles. Careful note should be made of the relationship of the remedy as indicated in the Materia Medica before making the next prescription.

Antidotal Relationship

Where untoward bad effects are observed after the administration of a remedy it may be necessary to antidote that remedy. This may be achieved by giving a remedy which matches the symptoms now apparent, and the remedy is usually found to be one which has a similar action to that first prescribed.

SPEEDY PRESCRIBING

It is sometimes necessary to treat a patient quickly, e.g. as a result of a sudden injury, bad news, or an unexpected disaster on a holiday. It is helpful if some remedies can be memorised that apply generally to these causes; causes we may call 'acquired' because they do not strictly belong to or involve the person's temperament or nature. The list given below sets out some of the causes most likely to be met with and the remedies that could be administered safely in low potencies.

Anger:	Arn., Bry., Cham., China., Gels., Nux.v.
Bad Eggs: (eating)	Carbo.v.
Bad Fat: (eating)	Ars., Carbo.v.
Bad Fish: (eating)	All.c., Arbo.a., Carbo.v.
Bad Food: (eating)	Carbo.v.
Bad News: (hearing)	Gels.
Bad Water: (drinking)	All.c., Crotal.h.
Bathing, cold:	Mag.phos.
Bee-sting:	Ledum

Bereavement:	Ignatia
Bites:	Hypericum, Ledum
Dog-bites:	Hydrophob.
Blood-poisoning:	Pyr.
Bones, injuries to:	Ruta, Symph.
Bruises:	Arn. Led., Ruta.
Burns and Scalds:	Urtica Urens.
Coffee, abuse of:	Nux.v.
Cold, with damp:	Dulc.
Cold, dry winds:	Acon., Hep.
Damp. cold weather	Gels.
Damp, cold winds, exposure to	All.c., Calc.c.
Damp sheets:	Rhus.t.
Damp warm weather:	Carbo.v.
Dentition:	Cham., Mag.Phos.
Depressing Emotions:	Gels.
Eating, excess in:	Bry., Nux.v.
Emotions, depressing:	Gels.
pleasurable, effects of:	Coff.
Examination funk:	Anac.,Gels.
Eyes, Inuries to:	Aconite.
Eyes over-strain:	Ruta.
Fat:	Carbo.v., Ipec., Puls.
Fear:	Acon.
Feet wetting:	Puls.
Fractures:	Ruta., Symph.
Fruit:	Ars., China.
Grief:	Ars., Ign.
Head, blow on:	Hypericum.
Head, getting wet:	Bell., Rhus.t.
Ice-cream:	Puls.
Nerves, injury to:	Hypericum.
News, bad:	Gels.
Pastry:	Puls.
Punctured wounds:	Hypericum, Ledum.
Riding in carriage:	Cocc.
Storms:	Gels., Phos.
Sun: (too much)	Acon., Bell., Gels., Glon.

HOMOEOPATHIC REMEDIES

In dealing with the actual remedies it will be necessary for you to observe carefully certain rules. These may appear to be simple and even unimportant but we can assure you that they are of utmost importance. This will be evident to those students who have learnt through this course and appreciate the very delicate nature of the Homoeopathic medicines especially in their higher potencies or attenuations.

Rule 1:   Remedies should never be stored in the light, particularly bright sunlight, or near any strong smelling soaps, powders or liquids.

Rule 2:   Remedies should not be changed from one bottle to another unless the bottle is first sterilised (i.e. boiled for 20 minutes in a pan of water). This will ensure that the vibrations of the remedies are not disturbed. Impress on patients that they must not change their remedies from the bottles or boxes in which they receive them, to others which for them may be more convenient. If pills must be taken during a day when travelling, for instance, the requisite number should be tipped from the bottle into a clean envelope or piece of clean paper.

Rule 3:   If several remedies are being prepared for different patients, the hands should be washed between handling each remedy, under running water.

Rule 4:   Vessels in which medicines may have been dissolved for easy administration to a patient, and spoons which may have been used to measure doses *must* be boiled for 20 minutes in clean water before being used for other medicines or purposes.

The Homoeopathic remedies are prepared (potentised) from the mother tincture in the case of herbs and plants and this is known by the sign φ. In some cases treatment is effected by the use of the mother tincture when 10 or 15 drops, according to the remedy, are put into a small glass of water.

The potentised remedies are obtainable in pilules, tablets, granules, powders or liquids. You will find that the pilules are for the greater part the most convenient to use, but there will be occasions when tablets will be preferable and on others, granules or powders. It will make no difference to the value of the medicine itself but the different types of vehicle may have important psychological effects on a patient. Thus while it is sometimes advised to give 3 pills there is no real advantage as it is always the quality of the remedy that is important and not the amount taken.

DIET

Like Homoeopathy, diet is very individual and 'One man's meat is another man's poison'.

When treating patients with Homoeopathic remedies however, care should be taken regarding the diet of the patient, and advice given accordingly.

Samuel Hahnemann said very definitely that the correct food helped the remedies to work more quickly and effectively, and therefore the following remarks should be of interest to all students.

There is so much that is artificial in our foodstuffs today that it is essential to advise patients to eat as much 'Whole Food' as possible.

Compost-grown wheat flour (stone-ground) should be substituted for all bread and white flour products. 'Bread is the Staff of Life' but it has been proved that white bread contributes towards ill health and gives animals hysteria.

White sugar sweetens but leaves an acid reaction in the system often contributing to poor digestion.

A more crude form of sugar is molasses, the first pressing from the cane. This is full of valuable mineral salts including quantities of potassium and calcium and is of great value to those who suffer from inveterate constipation and digestive disorders.

A natural sugar is, of course, honey. A *pure* comb honey applied to wounds and ulcers will act as an antiseptic and powerful healing agent — but an application of blended honey has been found to increase the inflammation.

Generally speaking it is wise to advise plenty of salads, conservatively cooked vegetables and fresh fruit; fish, eggs, meat (preferably lamb) and poultry should be taken in moderation; good wholemeal bread and butter.

Peppermint (including that in toothpaste) should be avoided, also camphor, menthol, inhalents, disinfectants and all strong smelling cosmetics and perfumes. These will interfere with the delicate vibrations of the Homoeopathic remedies and thus spoil their effective action in the cure of disease.

Milk should be taken in moderation and unpasteurised milk bottled on the farm should be purchased if possible. Freshly made weak tea should be taken in moderation; China tea is much better than Indian. Fruit drinks made from fresh fruit should be recommended; also bran tea flavoured with fruit juices. Dandelion coffee can replace ordinary coffee and this is excellent for liver and kidneys.

One last word of advice which has proved many times to be valuable in the treatment of disease. Always enquire into the kind of vessels patients use for cooking. Homoeopathy has proved that many patients are definitely allergic to the poisoning effects of aluminium; when aluminium cooking pots have been replaced by stainless steel or enamel cooking pots the patients have responded more rapidly to the medicines prescribed and their cure has been considerably hastened.

With regard to specific diets for particular diseases you must always bear in mind the patient you are treating, his circumstances of home or business life. He is an individual and his diet must therefore be decided on the same principles.

THE HOMOEOPATHIC LAY PRACTITIONER

In this final lesson it is fitting that we draw your attention to one or two important points. Each student has his own reasons for studying Homoeopathy. Many wish only to learn more about this system of medicine to help those about them towards better health; to be able to treat in emergency those acute ailments which beset all members of a family at times, and to act in the knowledge that they are giving the right treatment until the Homoeopathic Physician arrives.

Those who unfortunately do not have an Homoeopathic Physician nearby — and there are many — are thrown on their own resources and feel compelled to make a deeper study so that they can with reasonable confidence treat ailments which do not assume too grave a character.

On the other hand, there are some students who, in their firm belief of Homoeopathic principles and in their desire to see Homoeopathy spreading, will extend the range of their treatments possibly building up a lay practice over a period of time. To these students especially the following remarks are addressed.

Let us review briefly some of the considerations which must be borne in mind. We believe that in this country, legally there are no diseases which may not be treated by a lay practitioner, but there are a number of diseases listed in the Pharmacy and Medicines Act 1941, for which *one must not claim cures*. This applies to both the written and the spoken word. One must, therefore, never make a claim for 'specified treatment' or any 'particular medicine' in the treatment of these diseases.

The wording of the Act at the time of going to press, is we believe as follows:

'Subject to the provisions of this Act, no person shall take part in the publication of any advertisement referring to any article, or articles of any description, in terms which are calculated to lead to the use of that article or articles of that description for the purpose of the treatment of human beings for any of the following diseases, namely, Bright's disease, cataract, diabetes, epilepsy or fits, glaucoma, locomotor ataxia, paralysis or tuberculosis:

'Provided that this sub-section shall not apply to an advertisement published by a local authority, or by the governing body of a voluntary hospital, or by any person acting with the sanction of the Secretary of State or the Minister of Health.'

The Act also contains a section regarding the advertisement of articles of any description for the procuring of miscarriage in women, and cancer.

Venereal Disease may only be treated when and where there is no free treatment available through a local authority or hospital. In view of the present health service it would appear unlikely that there are many places in the British Isles so remote as not to possess such facilities.

All Infectious Diseases must be reported to the local health authorities. These include the following — Small-pox, cholera, diphtheria, membranous croup, erysipelas, scarlatina or scarlet fever, typhus, typhoid (enteric), relapsing, continued and puerperal fevers, tuberculosis, cerebro-spinal meningitis, anterior polio-myelitis, and other diseases in certain localities.

Specific diagnosis of a disease should be avoided by a lay-practitioner as inLaw a proof of 'wrongful diagnosis' might be subsequently considered to be 'negligence' if the wrong treatment has been persisted in. In any serious condition or where any of the diseases listed above seems to be indicated, it is always as well to have a confirmatory diagnosis made by a registered doctor, in fairness to both yourself and the patient.

We suggest that great care should be taken when dealing with serious ailments and owing to the possibility of a change in the law it is advisable to consult a Solicitor when in doubt.

Remember at all times that in your behaviour and in your treatment of a patient it is Homoeopathy that is being judged. Any action or negligence on your part which brings discredit to you, also brings discredit to this system of medicine, and that, we are sure, you would not wish. Dr. Roberts in his book *The Principles and Art of Cure by Homoeopathy* states 'When in doubt, DON'T'. May we endorse this remark when the good name of Homoeopathy may be at stake.

SUMMARY

In this our last lesson, it is fitting that we review briefly the basic principles of Homoeopathy which it has been our endeavour to teach you. *The principles are unchanging* and it is our hope that as a result of your studies you have so absorbed these basic pinciples that it will be your wish never to deviate from them. Let us then briefly summarise the teachings of Hahnemann in order to be sure that they are firmly established in our minds:

Homoeopathy is a system of medicine based on the principle Similia Similibus Curentur — Let likes be treated by likes. In order to be curative the remedy prescribed must be capable of exciting similar symptoms in the body to those of which the patient complains.

There are kinds and degrees of similarity so that even though the perfect similimum may not always be found, a near similar may nevertheless stimulate the patient towards cure.

The remedies used in Homoeopathic practice have been thoroughly tested and their range of action established by being proved on healthy persons. The Homoeopathic practitioner, therefore, knows exactly what results to expect from the medicine when he prescribes it according to Homoeopathic principles.

The Homoeopathic Materia Medica is made up of the records of drug provings, supplemented by histories of poisonings and information derived from successful treatment, i.e. clinical evidence.

Case-taking is not only for the purpose of ascertaining a diagnosis but also to elicit the symptoms of each individual patient, both mental and physical, as they differ from the normal.

Symptoms have degrees of value for the purpose of making a prescription. General symptoms are of greater value than particular symptoms. Of the General symptoms those pertaining to the Mind rank the highest.

The remedy is selected by careful comparison of the characteristic totality of symptoms of the individual with that of drugs. The drug which is most homoeopathic is that one which is capable of producing symptoms most similar to that of the condition present.

The remedy finally selected for a patient must be the true similimum or that which most nearly covers the totality of symptoms. Its action should be carefully observed and no other remedy given until the remedial effect is exhausted.

The dose should be repeated only when improvement ceases and symptoms return to their original form. The interval between doses is governed by the severity of the case and whether the condition is acute or chronic. The remedy should be changed only when improvement ceases and/or symptoms change.

Improvement is evidenced by an increased sense of comfort and naturalness in the feelings of the patient. He feels better himself though his pains may be aggravated.

Cure takes place from above downward; from within outward; from an important organ to a less important organ; symptoms disappear in the reverse order of their appearance, the first to appear being the last to disappear. The return of old symptoms in a chronic case may, therefore, be taken as a sign of incipient cure.

In order to understand and appreciate the Homoeopathic system of medicine and the principles on which it operates, it is essential to know something about life — what it is and how it operates in animal and human bodies. Hahnemann postulated it is the Vital Force that animates a living body and maintains it in health. An interruption of its activity results in disease becoming manifest, while a total suspension results in death. This Vital or Life Force is dynamic in nature, possessing the power to create, organise, build and maintain living animal and human bodies in organic physical matter. Every process of life works from seed to organism, from the centre to the circumference, from within outwards. Homoeopathic remedies have a similar action and are thus in conformity with this great natural law.

Chapters 3—7, 11, 16—21, 31—35 of Roberts' *The Principles and Art of Cure by Homoeopathy* should now be read and studied.

TEST PAPER No. 12

These questions should be answered only when the student feels confident that the lesson has been mastered. There should be no reference to books as this would defeat the object.

1. If a patient complained of feeling unwell following an accident, what is the first remedy you would think of for him?

2. If a patient complained of catching many colds, which went on to the chest, how would you deal with the case? What questions would you ask and what medicines would you prescribe?

4. Name five symptoms which point to Psora.

BIBLIOGRAPHY

Some of the most useful and valuable books for continued study and use are:

A COMPARISON OF THE CHRONIC MIASMS by Phyllis Speight

A DICTIONARY OF PRACTICAL MATERIA MEDICA (3 volumes) by Dr. J.H. Clarke

A SONG OF SYMPTOMS by Patersimilias

CHRONIC DISEASE by Dr. S. Hahnemann

CLINICAL REPERTORY by Dr. J.H. Clarke

CONDENSED MATERIA MEDICA by Dr. C. Hering

HOMOEOPATHIC DRUG PICTURES by Dr. M.L. Tyler

HOW TO USE THE REPERTORY by Dr. G.I. Bidwell

LEADERS IN HOMOEOPATHIC THERAPEUTICS by Dr. E.B. Nash

LECTURES ON HOMOEOPATHIC MATERIA MEDICA by Dr. J.T. Kent

LECTURES ON HOMOEOPATHIC PHILOSOPHY by Dr. J.T. Kent

MATERIA MEDICA OF THE NOSODES by Dr. Allen

MATERIA MEDICA PURA by Dr. S. Hahnemann

REPERTORY by Dr. J.T. Kent

THE CHRONIC MIASMS by Dr. Allen

THE ORGANON by Dr. S. Hahnemann

VACCINOSIS by Dr. J.C. Burnett

The small books by Dr. J. Compton Burnett are well worth serious study. they include ENLARGED TONSILS.

FISTULA, GOLD, GOUT, LIVER, NATRUM MURIATICUM and TUMOURS.

Kent's REPERTORY is the best but it needs skill in handling. Bidwell's work, mentioned above, is helpful in this respect.

You are reminded that although you have read many extracts from THE ORGANON a complete study should be made of this work together with THE MATERIA MEDICA PURA and CHRONIC DISEASES by Hahnemann.

SPECIMEN ANSWERS

Test Paper No. 1
1. The Law of Similars — Simila Similibus Curentur.

2. Because pathological changes are the end product of disease. If the patient as a whole is treated he will, in time, lose all symptoms of sickness, providing he is curable.

3. Because the most similar remedy will give the healing processes of the body the boost they need to cure the patient.

Test Paper No. 2
1. Acquired and inherited. Acquired diseases from direct contamination with epidemic and endemic diseases. Inherited diseases are those which develop according to the idiocyncrasies of the patient.

2. In order that we can be sure any symptoms exhibited after taking the substance to be proved come from the symptoms of sickness of the prover and are not symptoms of the prover.

3. Terror; unreasonable fears; restlessness; suddenness of the appearance of symptoms. All symptoms worse cold, dry winds.

Test Paper No. 3
1. From above downwards (i.e. from shoulder to wrist). From within outward (this happens when there is a skin eruption, an attack of diarrhoea, vomiting etc). Symptoms disappear in the reverse order of their appearance (the last symptom is the first to go and the first is the last one to disappear).

2. The higher potencies should be given in chronic disease providing the vitality of the patient is strong enough and there is little or no organic change.

3.   Redness — heat, intense burning.

4.   Arnica should always be used after an accident as there is usually bruising of the soft parts and it is important to remove the shock which always follows. Arnica should always be used when a patient cannot sleep because of overtiredness caused by hard physical work.

5.   Hypericum should be given when a person suffers great pain after shutting his fingers in a door. The nerve endings suffer bruising and sometimes damage and hypericum deals with this and removes the pain.

Test Paper No. 4

      Acute conditions do not, as a rule, last very long. They attack, get worse and then there is always a tendency towards recovery. Chronic conditions, on the other hand, progress, sometimes very slowly, and there is no tendency towards recovery. The patient's vital force cannot control these diseases and they can be cured only by proper treatment.

2.   Psora, Syphilis and Gonorrhoea (Sycosis).

3.   Deep acting remedies that could affect the whole of man's economy. Remedies which act from the centre to the circumference.

4.   Restlessness. Intense burning but pains better by heat. Great and sudden prostration. Intense thirst but drinks little at a time.

Test Paper No. 5

      The deep-acting psoric remedies working from the centre to the circumference would in all probability bring out an eruption on the skin.

2.   A skin eruption is the manifestation of something wrong in the economy and ointments must never be applied as this would only push back into the system the poisons which are trying to come out. Headaches, flatulence, slight diarrhoea may also come to the surface — they should not be treated as they will disappear in a few days — they are but aggravations from the medicines.

3.   The classical child needing sulphur looks as though he needs a wash although he has just had one! His hair is lank and untidy; his clothes are dirty and often torn and he doesn't seem to notice. His eyes, ears and lips often look very red. This child will come into the room and collapse into a chair, especially mid-morning, and demand food. He often has odd spots, herpes, or an eruption somewhere on the skin.

Test Paper No. 6

1.   A nightly aggravation of all complaints. Destruction of tissue. Ulcerations including varicose ulcers. Sudden and severe diarrhoeas. Mentality slow, stubborn, sullen, stupid, suspicious. Menstrual troubles relieved by the outbreak of an ulcer. Destruction of nasal bones.

2.   Overgrowth of tissue — warts. Rheumatism and arthritis. Chronic catarrh. Thickening of skin and nails. Diseases of the sexual organs.

3.   Repeated vaccinations.

4.   Vaccinal poisons. Tea.

Test Paper No. 7

1.   Psora combined with syphilis.

2.   When a patient is suffering from all these symptoms the case must be taken and looked at very carefully in order that the active miasm at that time may be treated. As treatment progresses another miasm will show up and then that will have to be treated and so on.

3.   A nosode is a medicine made from morbid or disease products. A nosode may be used when the indicated remedy brings no good results. Often there is a barrier which the nosode will remove and then the constitutional remedy will do its job. Also, a nosode may be given when there is a family history of one of the chronic diseases, or when symptoms in the patient suggest a certain disease.

4.   There is very great sensitivity mentally but especially physically, to a draught of air, to least touch and to pain which sometimes becomes intolerable and causes the

patient to faint. Great tendency to suppurations. The slightest scratch or injury suppurates.

Test Paper No. 8

1.   We should learn all we can from the patient as they come in. A mental note should be made of things like their handshake, how they walk, how they are dressed and how they sit down. A great deal can be learned in this way before the actual serious talking begins.

2.   A young man asks for help for a hard and painful cough. He said that it started after he had walked home from work in a very cold wind. It was worse coming into a warm room from outside and he always held his chest as this seemed to ease the pain. He liked to be out in the open air. He had a good appetite but always had a lot of wind after meals which relieved a full feeling. He was thristy and drank a lot as his mouth was always dry. He was very irritable. Also very anxious but when he went out for a walk he felt better. This is a good picture of Bryonia.

3.   Avoid asking questions where the answer can be 'yes' or 'no'. Avoid trying to fit a remedy into the symptoms of the patient before the case has been taken fully. Avoid being biased and keep an open mind until all the pros and cons have been weighed up and the remedy picture emerges.

4.   Worse all movement. Worse dry cold winds. Better pressure. Dryness of mucous membranes.

Test Paper No. 9

1.   *General* symptoms are those that relate to the patient as a whole, when he says, 'I feel. . .'
     Mental symptoms are those which affect the will, under-standing and memory. When strongly marked they often supply the key to the prescription.
     Particular symptoms are those which are applicable to some part of the patient but are of least value when assessing the case.

2.   It is wrong to prescribe on particular symptoms as this would be treating an effect and not getting to the cause of the trouble which is sealed in the patient's economy.

3.   Lycopodium China and Carbo veg., are the three great
      'wind' remedies.
4.   Complaints are worse from 4 to 8 p.m.
      Complaints are right-sided or move from right to left.
      Patient is hungry but a little food soon causes a feeling of
      fullness and distension.
      Better warm drinks. Worse cold food and drink.

Test Paper No. 10
Mrs X aged 46 years.
Headaches constant:
   Worse lying.
   Occipital pain, sense of pressure.
Dizziness and dimness of vision.
Difficult breathing when ascending stairs.
   When leaning back.
Sighs much recently.
Sleep good at night, but tired in the morning.
Wants to sleep all the time;
   worse after eating.
Hungry, but easily satisfied.
No thirst
Flatus considerable.
Very restless.
Sadness from music.
Memory poor.
Speech stuttering recently.
Concentration difficult.
Imagines she sees things running across the floor, mice etc.
Thinks of nothing but death.
Homesick, whenever away visiting.
Irritable and cross.
Sensitive to noise.
Desires company.
Better in open air; must have it.
Very sensitive to tight collars, and tight clothing anywhere.
Urination frequent; copious,
   worse when on her feet.
Menstrual period irregular; delayed, at times two or three
months.

Flow copious 3 or 4 days.
Discharge very dark, strong odour, excoriating, during latter
part of period.

The most important symptoms is 'Imagines she sees things
running across the floor, mice etc.' and so we take the rubric
Delusions in the repertory and use the remedies that appear in
black type and italic only.

Another exercise is to repertorize this case which worked out
to Lycopodium and this cured.

Test Paper No. 11

1.   In acute disorders.

2.   a. That the remedy is correct but the vital organs have
      been affected which slows up improvement, or a cure is not
      possible.
      b. The remedy is correct.

3.   When the patient is improving NEVER repeat until
      improvement comes to a halt and the same symptoms
      start to return. If new symptoms arise then another
      remedy must be found to match them.

4.   A patient needing Silica is usually rather timid, and a
      person who gets het up anticipating events.
      He feels the cold very much, especially his head which he
      likes wrapped up even in bed.
      He is very susceptible to draughts and takes cold very
      easily.
      Every small wound suppurates.

Test Paper No. 12

1.   Arnica, because he would be suffering from shock.

2.   A full case history would have to be taken with special
      interest as to whether there was any history of T.B. or
      chest troubles in his immediate family, parents, grand
      parents, brothers or sisters.
      His constitutional remedy must be given but Bacillinum
      should also be thought of as this is the nosode which has an
      affinity with the lungs. It often does excellent work in
      strengthening them.

3.   You can only recognise the miasms from the symptoms of the patient and the uppermost will be recognised — again by symptoms. You may have a case where the sycotic miasm is uppermost, for instance the woman who has suffered a great deal from uterine troubles, has several warts and a fishy taste in her mouth. After treatment with sycotic remedies this may change and Psora may come to the top and she may then have a great itching of the skin, with hunger pains at night or mid-morning, with dry hot hands and feet — the soles burn.
Then a psoric remedy must be chosen.
After some time there will be another change and the Syphilitic miasm may come up or the Sycotic one may return. We can only remove the miasms 'in layers' rather like peeling an onion. It is a mistake to think that when a miasm has been treated and the symptoms change that it has been stamped out.

4.   a. A sinking feeling mid-morning.
b. Feels tired — flops into a chair or props himself against a wall.
c. Skin looks dirty often with an itching eruption.
d. Emotional disturbances make patient ill.
e. Hair lank, greasy, lustreless.